Prostaglandins and Fertility Regulation

Advances in Reproductive Health Care

(1984/85)

E. S. E. Hafez: Series Editor

LHRH and Its Analogs: Contraception and Therapeutic Applications
H. Vickery, J. J. Nestor, Jr. and E. S. E. Hafez (editors)

Spontaneous Abortion
E. S. E. Hafez (editor)

Voluntary Termination of Pregnancy
E. S. E. Hafez (editor)

Biomedical Aspects of IUDs
H. Hasson, W. A. A. van Os and E. S. E. Hafez (editors)

Prostaglandins and Fertility Regulation
M. Toppozada, M. Bygdeman and E. S. E. Hafez (editors)

Male Fertility and Its Regulation
T. Lobl and E. S. E. Hafez (editors)

Advances in
Reproductive Health Care

Prostaglandins and Fertility Regulation

editors

M. Toppozada,
M. Bygdeman
and
E. S. E. Hafez

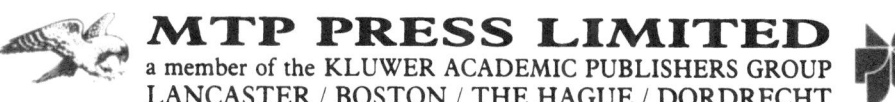

MTP PRESS LIMITED
a member of the KLUWER ACADEMIC PUBLISHERS GROUP
LANCASTER / BOSTON / THE HAGUE / DORDRECHT

Published in the UK and Europe by
MTP Press Limited
Falcon House
Lancaster, England

British Library Cataloguing in Publication Data

Prostaglandins and fertility regulation.—
  (Advances in reproductive health care)
  1. Human reproduction   2. Prostaglandins
  I. Toppozada, M.   II. Bygdeman, M.
  III. Hafez, E. S. E.   IV. Series
  612'. 6   QP251

   ISBN-13:978-94-010-8969-2   e-ISBN-13:978-94-009-5600-1
   DOI: 10.1007/978-94-009-5600-1

Published in the USA by
MTP Press
A division of Kluwer Boston Inc
190 Old Derby Street
Hingham, MA 02043, USA

Library of Congress Cataloging in Publication Data

Main entry under title:

Prostaglandins and fertility regulation.

  (Advances in reproductive health care)
  Includes bibliographies and index.
  1. Abortion.   2. Prostaglandins—Physiological effect.
3. Generative organs—Effect of drugs on.
I. Toppozada, M.   II. Bygdeman, M.   III. Hafez, E. S. E.,
1922–   . IV. Series.
RG734.P76 1984   618.8'8   84–7921

Typeset by Macmillan India Ltd, Bangalore.

Contents

CONTENTS

List of Contributors

J. J. AMY
Department of Gynecology/Andrology
  and Obstetrics,
Academisch Ziekenhuis, Vrije
  Universiteit Brussel,
Laarbeeklaan, 101, B-1090 Brussels,
BELGIUM

M. BYGDEMAN
Department of Obstetrics and
  Gynecology,
Karolinska Hospital,
10401, Stockholm 60, SWEDEN

N. J. CHRISTENSEN
Department of Obstetrics/Gynecology
  and Clinical Chemistry,
Karolinska Hospital, S-104 01,
Stockholm, SWEDEN

Z. R. GRAVES
The Department of Obstetrics and
  Gynecology,
Mount Sinai School of Medicine,
1 Gustave L. Levy Place,
New York, New York 10029, USA

K. GRÉEN
Department of Clinical Chemistry,
Karolinska Hospital, S-104 01,
Stockholm 60, SWEDEN

E. S. E. HAFEZ
Reproductive Health Center,
Medical University of South
  Carolina,
Department of Physiology,
171 Ashley Charleston, SC 29455, USA

R. W. HALE
Department of Obstetrics and
  Gynecology,
University of Hawaii, John A.
Burns School of Medicine,
Honolulu, Hawaii, USA

L. HAMBERGER
Department of Obstetrics and
  Gynecology,
University of Göteborg,
Sahlgren's Hospital, S-413 45,
Göteborg, SWEDEN

F. A. KIMBALL
Fertility Research,
The Upjohn Company, Kalamazoo,
MI 49001, USA

K. T. KIRTON
Fertility Research,
The Upjohn Company, Kalamazoo,
MI 49001, USA

W. KUHN
Department of Gynecology and
  Obstetrics,
University of Göttingen,
Humboldtallee 3, D-3400
Göttingen, FRG

H. KÜHNLE
Department of Gynecology and
  Obstetrics,
University of Göttingen,
Humboldtallee 3, D-3400
Göttingen, FRG

N. H. LAUERSEN
The Department of Obstetrics and
  Gynecology,
Mount Sinai School of Medicine,
1 Gustave L. Levy Place, New York,
New York 10029, USA

T. H. LIPPERT
Department of Obstetrics and
  Gynecology,
University of Tuebingen, D-7400,
Tuebingen, WEST GERMANY

LIST OF CONTRIBUTORS

V. LUNDSTRÖM
Department of Obstetrics and
  Gynecology,
Karolinska Hospital, S-104 01,
  Stockholm,
SWEDEN

A. NORSTRÖM
Department of Obstetrics and
  Gynecology,
University of Göteborg, Sahlgren's
  Hospital, S-413 45 Göteborg,
SWEDEN

W. RATH
Department of Gynecology and
  Obstetrics,
University of Göttingen, Humboldtallee
3, D-3400, Göttingen, FRG

S. D. SHARMA
Department of Obstetrics and
  Gynecology, University of Hawaii,
John A. Burns School of Medicine,
  Honolulu, Hawaii, USA

V. M. STEINMILLER
Department of Obstetrics and
  Gynecology,
University of Hawaii, John A. Burns
  School of Medicine, Honolulu,
  Hawaii,
USA

P. THEOBALD
Department of Gynecology and
  Obstetrics,
University of Göttingen,
Humboldtallee 3, D-3400, Göttingen,
FRG

J. TJUGUM
Department of Obstetrics and
  Gynecology,
University of Göteborg, Sahlgren's
  Hospital, S-413 45, Göteborg,
SWEDEN

M. K. TOPPOZADA
Department of Obstetrics and
  Gynecology,
Faculty of Medicine, The University of
  Alexandria,
EGYPT

O. VESTERQVIST
Department of Clinical Chemistry,
Karolinska Hospital, S-104 01,
  Stockholm,
SWEDEN

L. WILHELMSSON
Department of Obstetrics and
  Gynecology,
University of Göteborg, Sahlgren's
  Hospital, S-413 45, Göteborg,
SWEDEN

Foreword

The role of prostaglandins in physiological events and pathological disorders related to human reproduction has been most actively investigated in the past decade. Their clinical use for fertility regulation, extensively evaluated, represents the most common clinical indication for the administration of these remarkable compounds. Thus, it is most appropriate to update the available information related to the use of prostaglandins in the regulation of human fertility to provide a background document for the benefit of clinicians and scientists. Invited experts of international reputation from various parts of the world have contributed, each in his own area of interest, to offer this book, which we hope will fill an existing gap.

M. T.
M. B.
E. S. E. H.

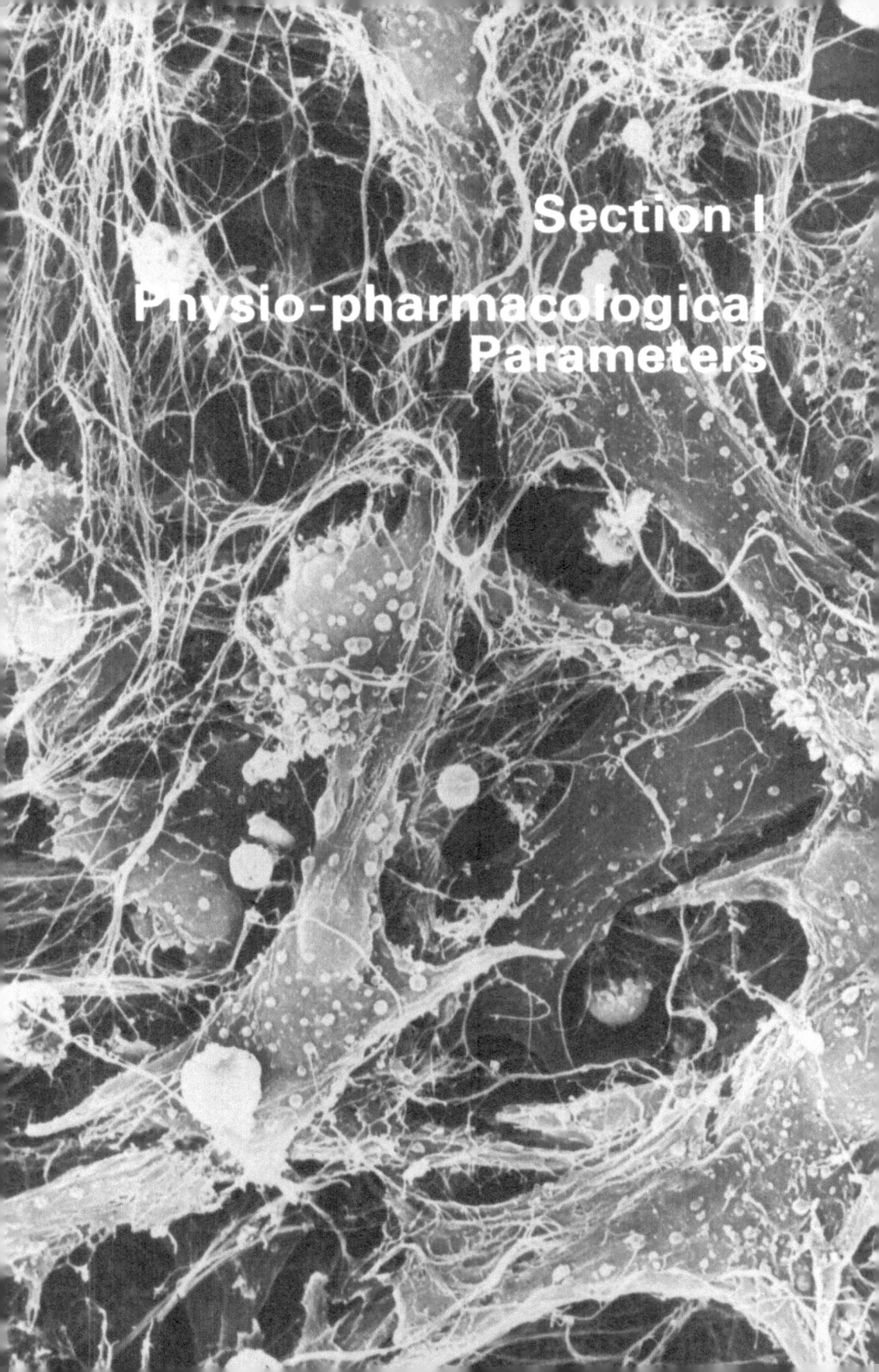

Section I
Physio-pharmacological Parameters

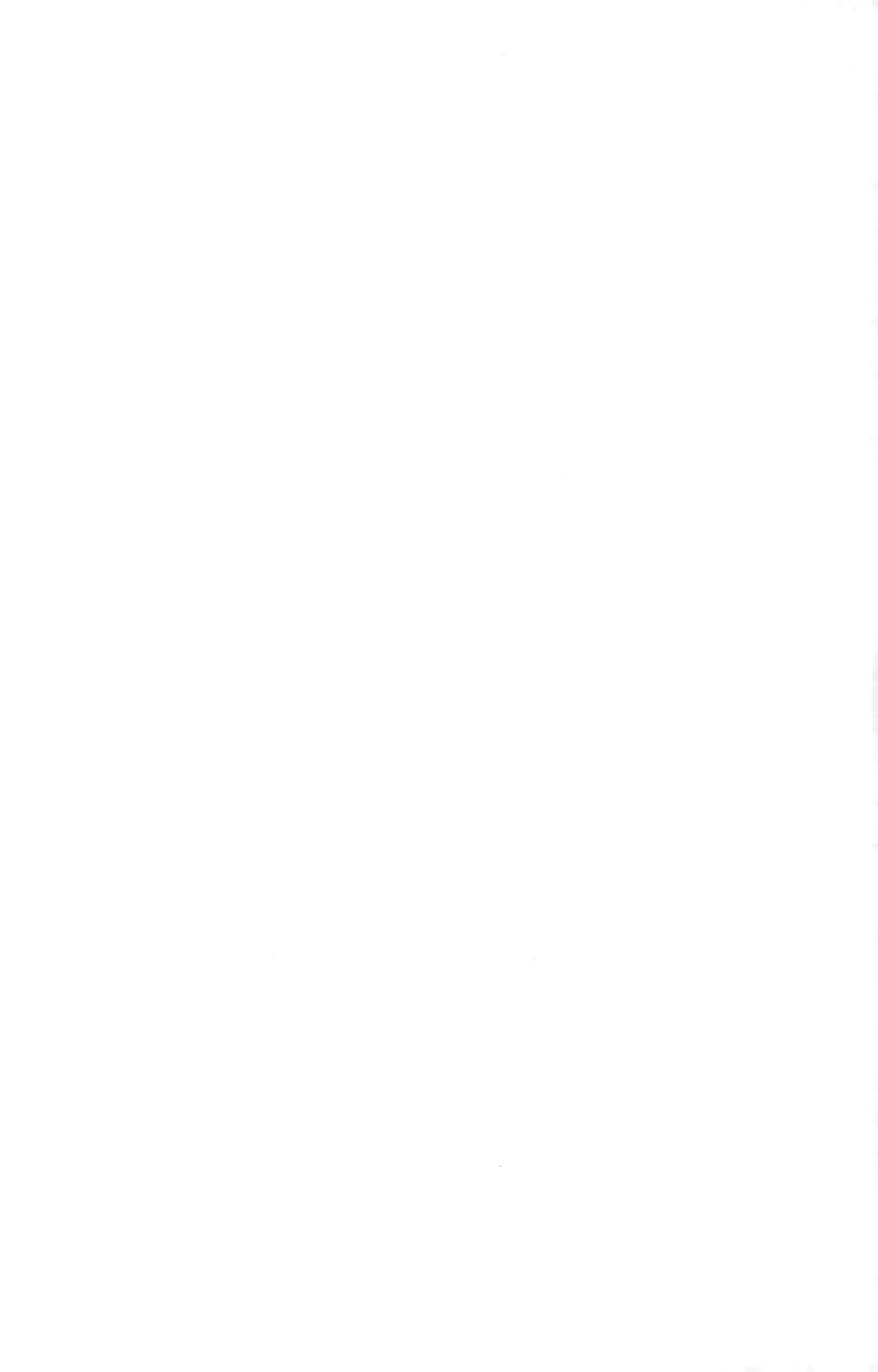

1
Potential for prostaglandin use in controlling human reproduction

K. T. KIRTON and F. A. KIMBALL

BACKGROUND

It was observed in 1930 that seminal plasma of a number of species contained very large amounts of substance(s) capable of altering uterine motility. These substances were subsequently demonstrated to be prostaglandins (PGs); this began the early and continued association of this group of compounds with reproduction. The activity was found to be associated with a fraction containing lipid-soluble acids, derived from prostanoic acid. Restrictions imposed by obscure sources and small amounts of material available for testing were initially impediments to their study. However, after some time and considerable effort, a cooperative venture by The Upjohn Company and scientists at the Karolinska Institute resulted in the isolation of compound in pure form from sheep vesicular glands. The structures of PGE_1 and $PGF_{1\alpha}$ were subsequently determined (Bergstrom et al., 1968; Bergstrom and Sjovall, 1957). Larger amounts of materials were then prepared which enabled biologists to investigate their properties more extensively in a number of tests.

Prostaglandins comprise one group of a series of structurally related compounds that make up the arachidonic acid cascade. These polyunsaturated fatty acids are metabolic products of cell membrane phospholipids, liberated through phospholipase activation in response to a diverse number of stimuli. They are extremely potent, and have a very short metabolic half-life in peripheral circulation. As a group, the prostaglandins are synthesized in very small amounts in response to a number of different types of stimuli and are found in almost all species. For the most part they are synthesized, have a physiologic action, and then are metabolized within the cell prior to being released into the general circulation. Therefore they are not hormones in the classical sense.

Their normal physiologic role has been difficult to determine, in a large measure because of their extreme potency, metabolic instability, widespread occurrence, and bioactivity (Hinman, 1972). Additionally, suppression of synthesis does not drastically impair an animal's body function. The prostaglandins have a number of properties that further contributed to the

3

challenge of their development as useful pharmacologic agents. The naturally occurring molecules are both chemically and metabolically unstable, inactivated and excreted very rapidly, and have a broad spectrum of pharmacologic actions. These properties dictated development of unique formulations and delivery systems to successfully develop their therapeutic potential (Karim, 1975). Examples are the intra-amniotic injection of $PGF_{2\alpha}$ where the compound is released slowly from a reservoir in a sustained manner, and the vaginal formulations which have advantages of an improved therapeutic ratio, potential of self-administration, and use of sustained-release preparations.

Mechanism studies in reproduction

Some of the early studies demonstrated a capacity for interruption of pregnancy in rodents and rabbits. Prostaglandin $F_{2\alpha}$ was active when administered by the subcutaneous route in early stages of gestation (Gutknecht et al., 1969). It was hypothesized that this was brought about through an inhibition of corpus luteum function (Pharriss, 1970). The mechanism was thought to be through alteration of the normal hemodynamics of the tissue. Prostaglandin $F_{2\alpha}$ has been shown to have vasoconstricting properties. This was in keeping with a hypothesis of luteolysis by an inhibition of venous blood flow. Extensive experimentation in many species of laboratory and domestic animals, as well as human clinical trials, followed. Significant species differences in sensitivity to prostaglandin-induced depression of corpus luteum function were demonstrated. Domestic animals have proven to be especially sensitive. Because of this, and the natural occurrence of prostaglandin in uterine tissue at the time of corpus luteum regression, it has been suggested that $PGF_{2\alpha}$ is the naturally occurring luteolytic factor in most sub-primate species (Goding, 1974). They are thought to play a role in corpus luteum function in some species, parturition, and endometrial sloughing during menses in primates. There is also a suggestion of effects on gamete transport.

An initial study in rhesus monkeys confirmed that $PGF_{2\alpha}$ was capable of terminating early stages of gestation; however, the mechanism was not obvious (Kirton et al., 1970). Since this prostaglandin was capable of stimulating the pregnant uterus, it could have been either through diminution of luteal function or by uterine stimulation. Stimulation of uterine smooth muscle is one of the most sensitive, repeatable biological responses to exogenous prostaglandins (Table 1.1). This was suggestive of therapeutically useful activity. It was determined that small variations of the molecular structure changed the relative potency significantly. In general, potencies were $E > F_\alpha > A > B$. Conversion to the 13,14-dihydro-15-keto metabolite significantly reduced the biopotency, as did beta-oxidation of the C_1 carbon side-chain. Chemical modifications of the molecule which retarded metabolic degradation enhanced in vitro activity (Kirton et al., 1976). More detailed studies were initiated to elucidate the mechanism of prostaglandin action on the uterus. It was determined that specific saturable binding sites for prostaglandins did exist in uterine tissue. The affinity of these binding sites was

4

Table 1.1 Uterine response to an acute intravenous injection of prostaglandin in rhesus monkeys

Compound	Amount injected (μg)	Δ Tone (mm Hg)
$PGF_{2\alpha}$	500	30
$15(S)15\text{-me-PGF}_{2\alpha}$	50	20
$15(S)15\text{-me-PGF}_{2\alpha}$	10	5
PGE_2	10	20
$15(S)15\text{-me-PGE}_2$	2	25

in keeping with the dose of prostaglandin necessary to stimulate the uterus (Table 1.2). In addition, the relative affinity of different structures was correlated with their uterine stimulating potency (Kimball and Kirton, 1977). Results of these studies and others indicate that the primary mechanism of pregnancy termination is directly on the uterus through stimulation of myometrial smooth muscle cell contractility. These studies have been confirmed, for the most part, in the human, and are thought to be one of the primary mechanisms of prostaglandin-induced human pregnancy termination.

Table 1.2 Relative affinities of prostaglandins as competitors of $[^3H]PGE_1$ binding in human myometrial low-speed supernatant and relative potencies of prostaglandins on rhesus uterine contractility *in vivo*

Name	Relative affinity[a]	Relative potency Pregnant[b]
A. PGE_1	100	10
PGE_2	80.2(98.9–65.0)	10
$PGF_{2\alpha}$	8.2(9.5–7.1)	1
PGA_1	2.8(3.6–2.1)	—
PGA_2	1.9(2.7–1.3)	0.5
PGB_1	0.9(1.3–0.6)	—
PGB_2	3.3(4.0–2.3)	0.2
PGD_2	none	< 0.2
B. 13,14-dihydro-PGE_1	18.4(27.2–12.0)	7
13,14-dihydro-15-keto-PGE_1	1.4(1.7–1.2)	1
15-keto-PGE_1	none	1
C. 15(S)-15-methyl-PGE_2	157.7(194.9–127.9)	100
15(S)-15-methyl-PGE_2 methyl ester	44.4(53.8–36.0)	—
15(S)-15-methyl-$PGF_{2\alpha}$ tham	6.0(7.0–5.2)	10
15(S)-15-methyl-$PGF_{2\alpha}$ methyl ester	1.6(1.9–1.3)	—

[a] 95% confidence interval in parentheses.
[b] Acute intravenous administration.

Delivery of prostaglandins

The development and experimentation with prostaglandins has been hampered by their instability and difficulty in designing suitable delivery systems.

The short biological half-life has dictated that these compounds be delivered either in constant infusions or in multiple dosing regimens. Only a relatively few of the activities are manifest after a single intramuscular or subcutaneous injection. The luteolytic activity in rodents and domestic animals is of this type (Karim, 1975). More common is the need for continuous dosing or multiple dose. For example, induction of labor at term is accomplished by intravenous infusion of PGE_2. More recent advances in formulation development for this indication are the use of orally or vaginally active tablets (Lange *et al.*, 1983). There has also been the development of gel formulations of PGE_2 which provide prolonged activity when delivered vaginally or endocervically (Mackenzie and Embrey, 1978).

Development of pharmaceutically useful preparations necessarily takes into account the physical and chemical properties of the compound. Prostaglandins as a group are considered unstable in the presence of high temperature, humidity, pH or certain ions (Bergstrom *et al.*, 1963). The instability of PGI_2 and PGE_2 has been well documented and has complicated both the design and interpretation of experimental results. Failure to replicate early results may have resulted, in part, from important differences in handling these sensitive compounds.

The experience of academic and clinical investigators has provided much information in the formulation and delivery of prostaglandins for *in vivo* and *in vitro* use. The unprecedented synthetic work in this field gave much to the understanding of the extreme lability of these molecules. Modifications in chemical structure have increased the stability of the parent molecule to enzymatic degradation. The introduction of methyl groups at carbon 15, 16 or 17 of the lower side-chain inhibits degradation by the 15-dehydrogenase enzyme (Bundy *et al.*, 1971). The shifting of the double bond or introduction of oxygen in the upper side-chain slows beta-oxidation (Samuelsson *et al.*, 1971). The modification of the pentane ring at carbon 9 or 11 may significantly reduce the level of conversion of PGE to PGA or PGB (Kimball *et al.*, 1979).

The development of long-acting formulations for prostaglandins has proceeded slowly because of their instability and their low effective doses. Vaginal formulations using PGE_2 for induction of labor have been reported for a number of years (Mackenzie and Embrey, 1977). These formulations gave clinically good results and were well received by the practitioner. However, until recently none of them was stable for long periods of time (18 months to 2 years). Recently some of these problems seem to have been solved. A second example is the use of polymer delivery systems. Clinical and animal studies using silicone devices containing 15-methyl-$PGF_{2\alpha}$ methyl ester showed the potential for this type of sustained delivery of prostaglandins (Greene and Gilling, 1979). These devices produced sustained blood levels of drug following an initial high level of release. It was this high level of prostaglandin which limited the clinical utility of the devices. Development of a more complex delivery system utilizing polymeric drug-releasing membranes demonstrates the potential for this type of approach (Roseman *et al.*, 1982). Further modification of this concept may lead to useful application of prostaglandins for several clinical uses.

6

Human clinical uses

A number of different clinical uses have been developed to the stage of marketed products in many locations throughout the world (Table 1.3). The original uses were with prostaglandin $F_{2\alpha}$ and prostaglandin E_2, both naturally occurring compounds, for either elective or therapeutic termination of pregnancy or to enhance delivery at term through either stimulation of the uterine muscle or preparation of the non-receptive cervix. Additional uses being developed at present are for the prevention or treatment of postpartum hemorrhage and treatment of severe toxemia of pregnancy. Prostaglandins are believed to be involved in a number of other physiologic processes associated with reproductive physiology. These include gamete transport in the female and male, ovulation, and pituitary function. However, these actions have not been developed as means of fertility control.

Two uses of PGE_2 in the term pregnant woman have become clinically important. The preparation and softening of the unfavorable cervix in those cases in which delivery is past due, or therapeutically desirable, has the potential for reducing the number of cesarean sections (Calder *et al.*, 1977). The activity of the prostaglandin appears to be principally on the uterine cervix, acting directly on the collagen matrix (Norstrom *et al.*, 1983). When the dose of PGE_2 is low and the drug is locally applied, the effect on the uterine muscle is frequently minimal. Labor may then develop spontaneously. When higher doses of PGE_2 are delivered the drug may also initiate uterine contractions and induce labor (Shepard *et al.*, 1979). This process may be completed with or without the use of oxytocin.

Table 1.3 Reproductive associated uses of prostaglandins, approved and under current development, in humans and domestic animals

Species	Use	
	Marketed	*Under development*
Human	Labor induction	Postpartum hemorrhage
	Second trimester abortion	Cervical dilatation/softening
		First trimester pregnant
	Death *in utero*	Prior to term delivery
		Non-pregnant
	Termination of abortion	Menses induction
	Failures by other means	Toxemia of pregnancy
Domestic animal	Estrus synchronization	
	Cattle	
	Horse	
	Induction of parturition	
	Pigs	
	Silent estrus	
	Cows	
	Horses	
	Parturition	
	Cows	
	Abortion	
	Cows	

Several large multicenter, multinational trials have been conducted to examine the utility of various prostaglandin analogs for use in the elective and therapeutic terminations of pregnancy. The results using 15(S)-15-methyl-$PGF_{2\alpha}$ THAM for interruption of second trimester pregnancies demonstrate the effectiveness of this type of therapy (Kajanoja et al., 1983). The procedure does result in a significant level of gastrointestinal side-effects. These can be reduced by aggressive premedication with antiemetic and antidiarrheals, or by a 12-hour treatment with laminaria prior to the prostaglandin therapy (Sharma et al., 1983). The benefit of the prostaglandin therapy compared to conventional intra-amniotic hypertonic saline is the non-invasive procedure which does not require routine use of surgical facilities. Later trials have used suppositories containing 15(S)-15-methyl-$PGF_{2\alpha}$ methyl ester for this same indication (World Health Organization, 1983). Ongoing trials are exploring the utility of prostaglandins for preoperative cervical dilatation and softening prior to suction curettage (Ganguli et al., 1977). These studies similarly demonstrate the efficacy of the compounds and the benefit of potential reduction in cervical trauma usually occurring as the result of forceful mechanical dilatation.

The use of potent prostaglandin analogs to interrupt very early pregnancy without the need of surgical intervention has been a long-standing clinical goal. The benefits to the patient of convenience, safety and privacy are parallel to the benefits to the community of lower medical costs and a reduced use of scarce and expensive surgical resources. The progress in this area has been slow – largely because of the need to administer these potent prostaglandin analogs for several hours in a way that does not result in an unacceptably high level of side-effects. Recent reports detailing the use of a PGE_2 analog in carefully selected patients treated at home demonstrates the potential for this type of therapy (Bygdeman et al., 1981). Further development will undoubtedly proceed at careful incremental steps.

Following early studies with prostaglandins a number of additional compounds were isolated which were proven to result from the complex arachidonic acid cascade. Like the original prostaglandins, many of these compounds also affect a number of different body processes. They also appear to have very complex interactions (Granström, 1983). The involvement of prostacyclin and thromboxanes in pregnancy has been suggested by several investigators (Kimball, 1983). These actions will continue to be explored for their medical utility.

Domestic animal use

The role of prostaglandins in the luteolytic process has been one of the most heavily studied of all areas in animal reproduction in recent years. The early suggestion that luteolysis is at least partially affected by local intraluteal circulatory changes continues to be studied (Pharriss and Kirton, 1969). The description of prostaglandin-specific binding sites in corpora lutea (Kimball, 1974) and their occurrence during the cycle (Kimball and Lauderdale, 1975) and in specific luteal cell types (Fitz et al., 1982) have further demonstrated the complexity of this mechanism. The equine and bovine corpora lutea are exceptionally sensitive to $PGF_{2\alpha}$ as a luteolytic agent. The demonstration of endogenous intrauterine production of $PGF_{2\alpha}$ during the latter part of the estrous cycle has given strength to the argument that $PGF_{2\alpha}$ is the natural luteolysin (Bartol *et al.*, 1981). It is not necessarily, however, the only factor involved in the cyclic demise of the corpus luteum in these species.

Prostaglandins have been developed for commercial use in domestic animal reproduction. Uses include synchronization of estrus, induction of therapeutic abortion and induction of parturition. Sheep, swine, cattle, and horses are species that have been investigated. The primary mode of action is probably inhibition of corpus luteum function, with a lesser role for the uterine stimulating activity.

Thus, the promise of the early studies has been borne out. These molecules have been shown to have a role in the normal physiology of the reproductive process and have been developed to a point where they are used in the pharmacologic control of fertility and treatment of obstetric problems. In addition, prostaglandins and their synthetic analogs have a number of additional potential uses which are continuing to be developed for the future.

References

Bartol, F. F., Thatcher, W. W., Bazer, F. W., Kimball, F. A.,Chenault, J. R., Wilcox, C. J. and Roberts, R. M. (1981). Effects of the estrous cycle and early pregnancy on bovine uterine, luteal and follicular responses. *Biol. Reprod.*, **25**, 759–776

Bergström, S. and Sjovall, J. (1957). The isolation of prostaglandins. *Acta Chem. Scand.*, **11**, 1086

Bergström, S., Carlson, L. A. and Weeks, J. R. (1968). The prostaglandins: a family of biologically active lipids. *Pharmacol. Rev.*, **20**, 1–48

Bergström, S., Ryhage, R., Samuelsson, B. and Sjovall, J. (1963). Degradation studies on prostaglandins. *Acta Chem. Scand.*, **17**, 2271–2280

Bundy, G., Lincoln, F., Nelson, N., Pike, J. and Schneider, W. (1971). Novel prostaglandin syntheses. *Ann. N Y Acad. Sci.*, **180**, 76–90

Bygdeman, M., Christensen, N. J., Gréen, K. and Zhery, S. (1981). Self administration of prostaglandin for termination of early pregnancy. *Contraception*, **24**, 45–52

Calder, A. A., Embrey, M. P. and Tait, T. (1977). Ripening of the cervix with extra-amniotic prostaglandin E_2 in viscous gel before induction of labor. *Br. J. Obstet. Gynaecol.*, **84**, 264–268

Fitz, J. A., Mayan, M. H., Sawyer, H. R. and Niswender, G. D. (1982). Characterization of two steroidogenic cell types in the ovine corpus luteum. *Biol. Reprod.*, **27**, 703–711

Ganguli, A. C., Gréen, K. and Bygdeman, M. (1977). Preoperative dilatation of the cervix by single vaginal administration of 15-methyl-$PGF_{2\alpha}$ methyl ester. *Prostaglandins*, **14**, 779–784

Goding, J. R. (1974). The demonstration that $PGF_{2\alpha}$ is the uterine luteolysin in the ewe. *J. Reprod. Fertil.*, **38**, 261–271

Granström, E. (1983). The prostaglandins, thromboxanes and leukotrienes. In: The importance of prostaglandins in obstetrics and gynecology. *Acta Obstet. Gynecol. Scand.*, Suppl. 113, 9–14

Greene, S. I. and Gilling, E. A. (1979). Postconceptional menses induction with a single dose of (15S)-15-methyl prostaglandin $F_{2\alpha}$ methyl ester in a silicone vaginal device. *Acta Therapeutica*, **5**, 143–153

Gutknecht, G. D., Cornette, J. C. and Pharriss, B. B. (1969). Antifertility properties of prostaglandin $F_{2\alpha}$. *Biol. Reprod.*, **1**, 367–371

Hinman, J. (1972). Prostaglandins. *Ann. Rev. Biochem.*, **41**, 161–178

Kajanoja, P. (1983). Induction of abortion by prostaglandins in the second trimester of pregnancy. A review. *Acta Obstet. Gynecol. Scand.*, Suppl. 113, 145–152

Karim, S. M. M. (1975). Advances in prostaglandin research. In Karim, S. M. M. (ed.). *Prostaglandins and Reproduction*. (Lancaster: MTP Press)

Kimball, F. A. (1974). Uterine prostaglandin binding proteins. *Prostaglandins*, **6**, 541

Kimball, F. A. (1983). Role of PGI_2 and other prostaglandins in pregnancy. In Lewis, P. J., O'Grady, J. and Moncoda, S. (eds.). *Prostacyclin and Pregnancy*. pp. 1–13. (London: Raven Press)

Kimball, F. A. and Kirton, K. T. (1977). Prostaglandins as antifertility agents. In Goldberg, M. E. (ed.). *Pharmacological and Biochemical Properties of Drug Substances*. pp. 373–386. (Washington, DC: American Pharmaceutical Association)

Kimball, F. A. and Lauderdale, J. W. (1975). Prostaglandin E_1 and $F_{2\alpha}$ specific binding in bovine corpora lutea: comparison with luteolytic effects. *Prostaglandins*, **10**, 313–331

Kimball, F. A., Bundy, G. L., Robert, A. and Weeks, J. R. (1979). Synthesis and biological properties of 9-deoxo-16,16-dimethyl-9-methylene-PGE_2. *Prostaglandins*, **17**, 657–666

Kirton, K. T., Kimball, F. A. and Porteus, S. E. (1976). Reproductive physiology: prostaglandin-associated events. In Paoletti, R. and Samuelsson, B. (eds.). *Advances in Prostaglandin and Thromboxane Research*, Vol. 2, pp. 621–625. (New York: Raven Press)

Kirton, K. T., Pharriss, B. B. and Forbes, A. D. (1970). Some effects of prostaglandins E_2 and $F_{2\alpha}$ on the pregnant rhesus monkey. *Biol. Reprod.*, **3**, 163–168

Lange, A. P., Westergaard, J. G., Secher, N. J. and Pedersen, G. T. (1983). Labor induction with prostaglandins. *Acta. Obstet. Gynecol. Scand.*, Suppl. **113**, 177–185

Mackenzie, I. R. and Embrey, M. P. (1977). Cervical ripening with intravaginal prostaglandin E_2 gel. *Br. Med. J.*, **2**, 1381–1384

Mackenzie, R. D. and Embrey, M. P. (1978). The influence of pre-induction vaginal prostaglandin E_2 gel upon subsequent labor. *Br. J. Obstet. Gynaecol.*, **84**, 657–661

Norström, A., Wilhelmsson, L. and Hamberger, L. (1983). Experimental studies on the influence of prostaglandins on the connective tissue of the human cervix uteri. *Acta Obstet. Gynecol. Scand.*, Suppl. **113**, 167–170

Pharriss, B. B. (1970). The possible vascular regulation of luteal function. *Perspect. Biol. Med.*, **13**, 434–444

Pharriss, B. B. and Kirton, K. T. (1969). Prostaglandin $F_{2\alpha}$: a new contraceptive approach. *Excerpta Med. Int. Congr.*, Ser No. 207, 2185

Roseman, T. J., Spilman, C. H., Tuttle, M. E., Lee, E. K. L. and Lonsdale, H. K. (1982). Membrane controlled delivery of prostaglandins. *Contraceptive Deliv. Syst.*, **3**, 460

Samuelsson, B., Granström, E., Gréen, K. and Hamberg, M. (1971). Metabolism of prostaglandins. *Ann. NY Acad. Sci.*, **180**, 138–163

Sharma, S. D., Hale, R. W. and Steinmiller, V. (1983). Intramuscular administration of 15(S)-15 methyl prostaglandin $F_{2\alpha}$ and laminaria insertion for termination of mid trimester pregnancy. *Contraceptive Deliv. Syst.*, **3**, 477

Shepard, J., Pearce, J. M. F. and Sims, C. D. (1979). Induction of labor using prostaglandin E_2 pessaries. *Br. Med. J.*, **2**, 108–110

World Health Organization (1983). Report of task force on the use of prostaglandins for fertility regulation. *Int. J. Gynaecol. Obstet.*, **21**, 159–165

2

Metabolism and pharmacokinetics of prostaglandin analogs in man

K. GRÉEN

The metabolism of naturally occurring primary prostaglandins was studied in several species during the 1960s. The investigations demonstrated that the metabolic degradation of these, biologically very potent, compounds was extremely rapid. The first step is an oxidation at carbon 15 in the prostaglandin molecule leading to biologically inactive metabolites which are then further degraded. The half-life in the human circulation of primary prostaglandins, e.g. PGE_2 and $PGF_{2\alpha}$, has been estimated to be 5–10 s (cf. Samuelsson *et al.*, 1975). The enzymes responsible for this rapid inactivation seem to appear in essentially all mammalian tissues (Samuelsson *et al.*, 1975; Änggård *et al.*, 1971). These studies led to efforts to synthesize prostaglandin analogs where this oxidation at carbon 15 was blocked, which created compounds with a longer duration of biological action than the natural prostaglandins.

Such analogs of major clinical interest in obstetrics and gynecology have been synthesized through introduction of methyl groups at carbons 15 and 16. Usually, administration of prostaglandins of the E-type is associated with fewer gastrointestinal side-effects than prostaglandins of the F-type. However, E-prostaglandins are potentially unstable because of the ring β-ketol, and therefore the ring structure has been modified in some analogs.

The objective of this article is to summarize some metabolic and pharmacokinetic data on four analogs, the structures of which have been designed along the lines indicated above; namely: 15(S)-15-methyl-$PGF_{2\alpha}$, 16,16-dimethyl-PGE_2, 9-deoxo-16,16-dimethyl-9-methylene-PGE_2 and 16,16-dimethyl-trans-Δ^2-PGE_1 methyl ester (Fig. 2.1). Of these, 16,16-dimethyl-PGE_2 so far seems to be too unstable in lipid base vaginal suppositories for large-scale clinical use, but the analytical metabolic studies on this analog have given valuable information for the development of other analogs.

The structures of the drugs covered in this article and the abbreviations that will be used are shown in Fig. 2.1. The metabolic studies have been performed with drug molecules labelled with tritium in the indicated positions. This means that two steps of β-oxidation of 16,16-dime-E_2 and 16,16-dime-t-Δ^2-E_1-me will lead to elimination of one tritium (at carbon 5) from the molecules and this will instead appear as tritiated water. In the presentation of the data

11

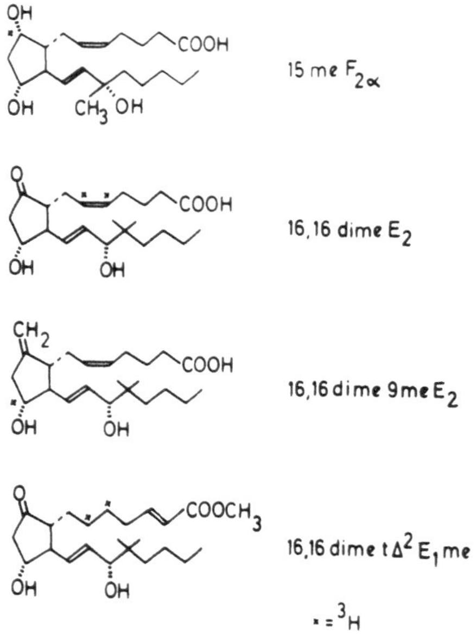

Figure 2.1 Structures of 15(S)-15-methyl-PGF$_{2\alpha}$ (15-me-F$_{2\alpha}$), 16,16-dimethyl-PGE$_2$ (16,16-dime-E$_2$), 9-deoxo-16,16-dimethyl-9-methylene-PGE$_2$ (16,16-dime-9-me-E$_2$) and 16,16-dimethyl-trans-Δ^2-PGE$_1$ methyl ester (16,16-dime-t-Δ^2-E$_1$-me)

on urinary excretion of radioactivity and metabolites this has been compensated for, in order to give directly comparable data on the four analogs.

INTRAVENOUS ADMINISTRATION OF LABELED ANALOGS

In a series of studies labeled analogs were injected into one antecubital vein and blood samples were drawn repeatedly from a contralateral antecubital vein (Hansson and Granström, 1977; Steffenrud, 1980, 1983; Dimov and Gréen, 1983). Plasma was isolated, and each sample analysed chromatographically for the amount of intact drug present in the circulation at each time, using either open-column reversed-phase partition chromatography or high-pressure reversed-phase partition chromatography. Somewhat different amounts of labelled drugs were injected (1.5–15 μg) but in view of the rapidity of metabolism it is unlikely that this has any major influence. As shown in Fig. 2.2 the most dramatic event is the very rapid hydrolysis of 16,16-dime-t-Δ^2-E$_1$-me to the free acid form. Already 1 min after injection about 50% of the administered amount (5 μg) has been transformed to the free acid, which then slowly disappears (Fig. 2.3). This is not unexpected since human plasma is known to contain esterases that rapidly hydrolyze prostaglandin methyl esters (Miller and Magee, 1974; Gréen and Bygdeman, 1976). Following administration of pharmacological amounts of this analog, the free acid is the major circulating form of this drug. From these studies of acutely injected drug it

12

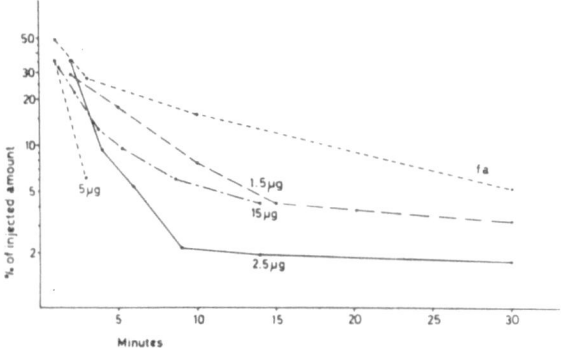

Figure 2.2 Disappearance of intact drugs from the circulation in percentage of given amount. $--.$, 15-me-$F_{2\alpha}$; $---$, 16,16-dime-E_2; ——, 16,16-dime-9-me-E_2; and. . . . , 16,16-dime-t-Δ^2-E_1-me (fa = free acid form)

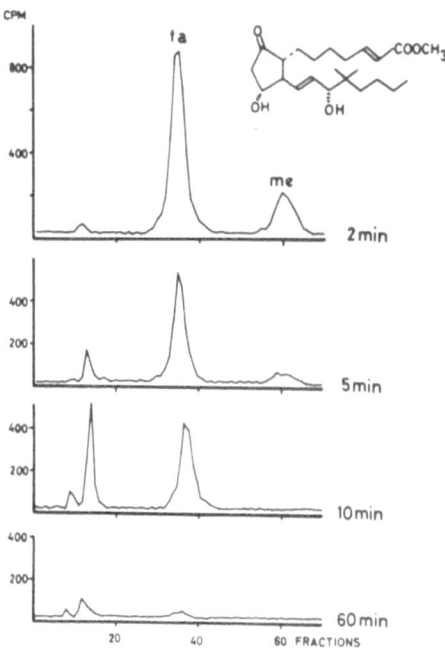

Figure 2.3 High-pressure reversed-phase chromatograms of plasma samples taken 2, 5, 10 and 60 min after i.v. administration of 5,6-[^{3}H]16,16-dime-t-Δ^2-E_1-me. Me = methyl ester, fa = free acid form of the analog

seems that 16,16-dime-9-me-E_2 disappears faster from the circulation than the other analogs, while the free acid of 16,16-dime-t-Δ^2-E_1-me is the slowest to disappear. This may not be entirely true since uptake of the analog in one or more tissues without noticeable metabolism, and then release thereof, may

13

occur in studies such as these. However, metabolic degradation of these compounds followed by release of metabolites into the circulation occurs quickly, as illustrated in Fig. 2.3 (cf. also Hansson and Granström, 1977). Only 2 min after i.v. injection of 5,6-[$^3H_2$]16,16-dime-t-Δ^2-E$_1$-me polar metabolites appear in plasma in addition to the methyl ester and free acid form of the drug.

Urinary excretion

Following i.v. injection of labeled analogs urine has been collected at intervals and the radioactivity and structures of urinary metabolites have been determined. The urinary excretion of radioactive metabolites (excluding tritiated water and including compensation for tetranor-metabolites of 16,16-dime-E$_2$ and 16,16-dime-t-Δ^2-E$_1$-me) is illustrated in Fig. 2.4. By far the largest urinary excretion is seen after injection of 15-me-F$_{2\alpha}$ while the smallest is seen after the 9-deoxo analog. The percentage of metabolites excreted in the urine is intermediary for the two other analogs. In cases given the 9-deoxo analog almost 60% of administered dose is excreted in the feces, indicating elimination via the bile. For comparison it is of interest to mention that about 90% of intravenously administered PGF$_{2\alpha}$ is excreted as metabolites in urine within 5 h (Granström and Samuelsson, 1969).

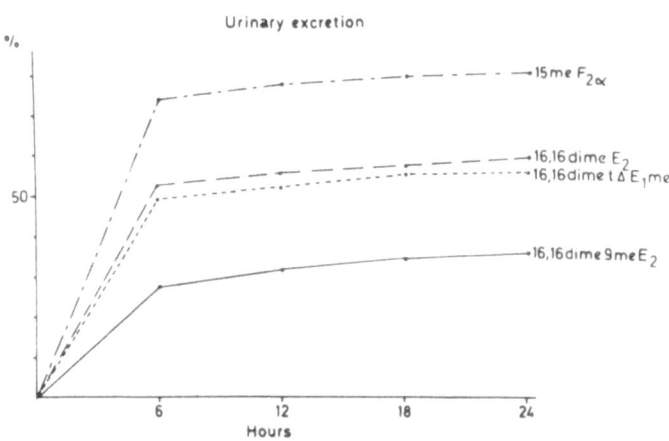

Figure 2.4 Percentage of administered amount excreted in the urine following i.v. injection of labeled 15-methyl-PGF$_{2\alpha}$ (15-me-F$_{2\alpha}$), 16,16-dimethyl-PGE$_2$ (16,16-dime-E$_2$), 9-deoxo-16,16-dimethyl-9-methylene-PGE$_2$ (16,16-dime-9-me-E$_2$) and 16,16-dimethyl-trans-Δ^2-PGE$_1$ methyl ester (16,16-dime-t-Δ^2-E$_1$-me)

URINARY METABOLITES

Some features are of enough general interest to be mentioned in this brief review. The structures of the analogs studied and proven points of attack on those molecules are shown in Fig. 2.5. The 15-hydroxy group is protected from

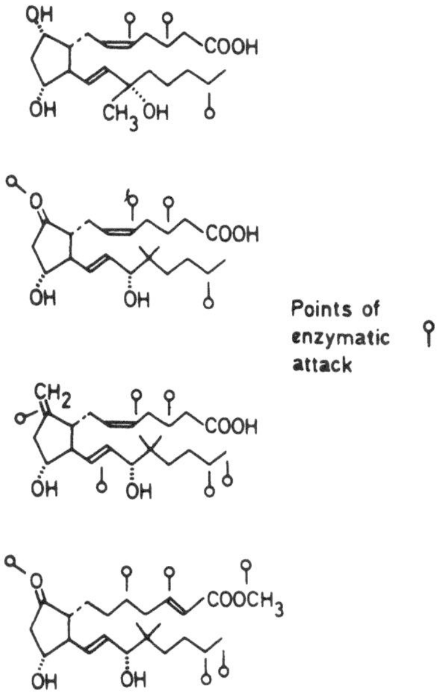

Figure 2.5 Structures of the analogs discussed in this article and proven points of enzymatic attacks on the molecules

oxidation in all four analogs. Such oxidation is the initial and very fast step in the metabolic degradation of natural primary prostaglandins. All four analogs can undergo two steps of β-oxidation and ω-oxidation at carbon 19 and/or 20. The oxygen at carbon 9 of the two E-analogs can be reduced to a hydroxyl group probably in β-position (unlike natural F-prostaglandins). The double bond of the methylene group at carbon 9 of the 9-deoxo analog can also be metabolically attacked, leading to several different ring structures (Fig. 2.6). This is an important metabolic route in the degradation of this analog since such metabolites constitute more than 20% of the injected radioactivity.

The major urinary metabolites of those four analogs are shown in Fig. 2.7. 15-methyl-PGF$_{2\alpha}$ and 16,16-dimethyl-PGE$_2$ are degraded via one or two steps of β-oxidation which leads to the major urinary metabolites. Some metabolites are ω-oxidized and perhaps some are excreted as conjugates (Hansson and Granström, 1977; Steffenrud, 1980). The ring ketone of the E-analog can also be reduced to a β-hydroxyl (cf. Fig. 2.5). Judging from the excretion pattern in urine it seems that 15-methyl-PGF$_{2\alpha}$ is less efficiently β-oxidized than 16,16-dimethyl-PGE$_2$ since as much as 40% of the F-analog is excreted as the dinor-metabolite as compared to 8% for the E-analog.

15-methyl-PGF$_{2\alpha}$ and 16,16-dimethyl-PGE$_2$ represent analogs where only one modification has been introduced into the molecules as compared to natural prostaglandins. These modifications have been directed towards blockage of the rapid enzymatic inactivation of the 15-hydroxy group and the metabolic degradation of those compounds is rather similar and follows routes earlier known for natural prostaglandins.

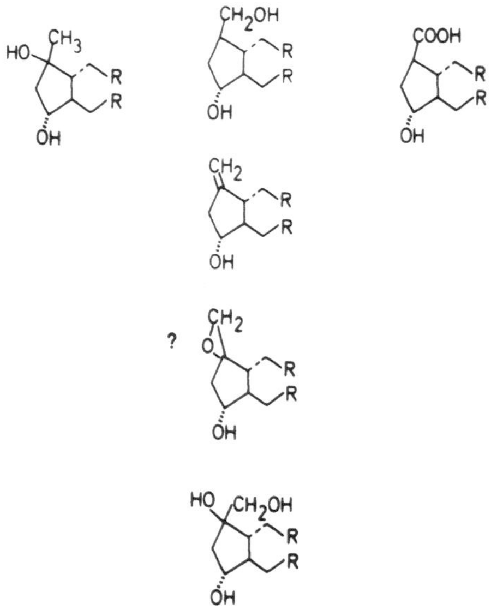

Figure 2.6 Ring structures of urinary metabolites of 9-deoxo-16,16-dimethyl-9-methylene-PGE$_2$

In the other two analogs, in addition to the 16,16-dimethyl-groups, another modification has been introduced into the molecules; namely a methylene group at C-9 and a Δ^2-trans double bond, respectively. The reason for using the methyl ester of 16,16-dimethyl-trans-Δ^2-PGE$_1$ is probably more of technical pharmaceutical nature (from a delivery system point of view) since it is rapidly hydrolyzed *in vivo*. These modifications alter the routes of metabolic inactivation prior to excretion dramatically, especially in the case of the 9-methylene analog. One obvious feature is the relatively small part of the administered amount of 9-deoxo-16,16-dimethyl-9-methylene-PGE$_2$ that is excreted into the urine as compared to the feces (Fig. 2.4). The explanation for this is found through analyses of the structures of the urinary metabolites (Fig. 2.7).

There is no single *major* metabolite found, as it is observed for the other analogs. Instead there is a wide variety of metabolites that has undergone considerable metabolic degradation but several of those are also to a great extent excreted in the form of conjugates (77% of urinary metabolites; Steffenrud, 1983). Most of these products are conjugates of glycine or glutathione. Such conjugations are known to occur particularly in the liver. Probably a large part of such metabolites is excreted via the bile leading to a low excretion of metabolites in the urine. The enzymatic attack on the double bond at C-9 is of special biochemical interest. Such degradation leads partly to a dihydrodiol and conjugates thereof, probably through an epoxide intermediate (Fig. 2.6).

The metabolism of 16,16-dimethyl-trans-Δ^2-PGE$_1$ is under study (Dimov

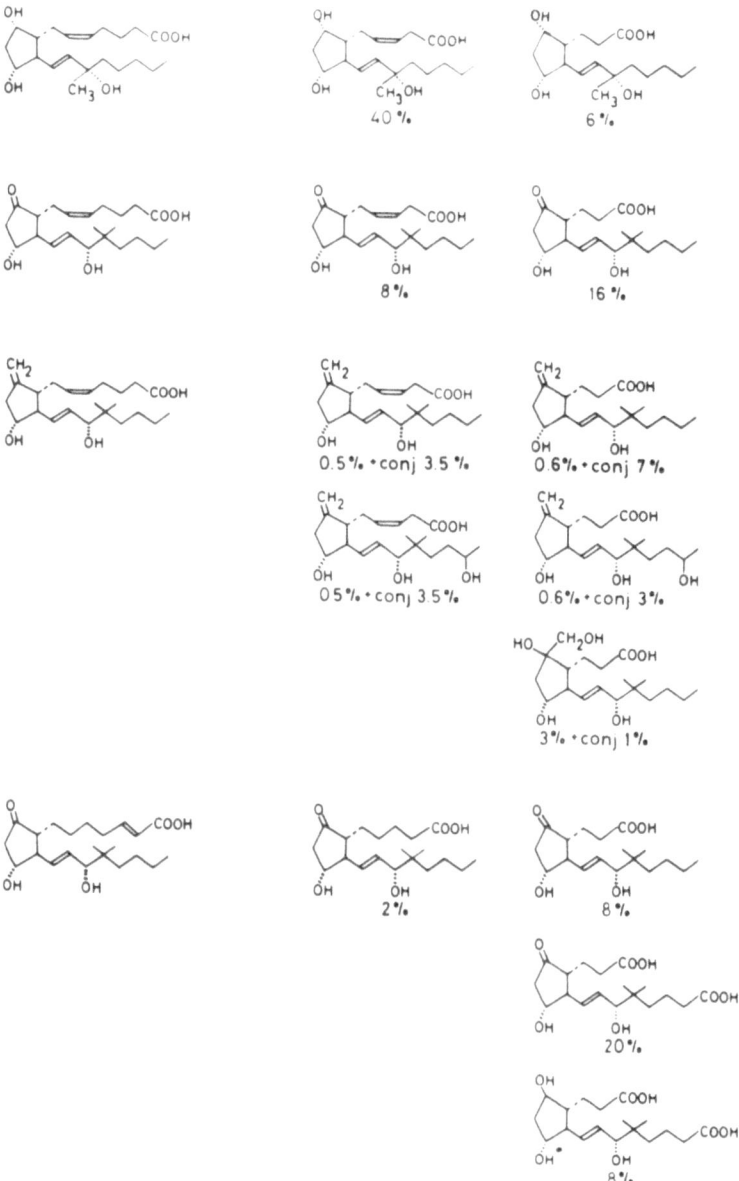

Figure 2.7 Structures of the four analogs and their major urinary metabolites. Figures in percentages refer to administered amount

and Gréen, 1983). The major urinary metabolite, 20% of the administered amount, is formed through two steps of β-oxidation and ω-oxidation to a dicarboxylic acid (Fig. 2.7). Relatively small amounts of metabolites from this analog are also excreted in the form of conjugates. Thus this analog is metabolized in a way similar to 16,16-dimethyl-PGE_2 in contrast to the 9-methylene analog.

THERAPEUTICAL PLASMA LEVELS

The plasma levels necessary for induction of abortions are also quite different for the four analogs. Figure 2.8 shows the plasma levels following administration of a single vaginal suppository containing 1 mg of 15-methyl-$PGF_{2\alpha}$ methyl ester, 16,16-dimethyl-PGE_2 or 16,16-dimethyl-trans-Δ^2-PGE_1 methyl ester or 30 mg of 9-deoxo-16,16-dimethyl-9-methylene-PGE_2. Such treatment gives rise to plasma levels enough for induction of first or second trimester abortions, but are maintained for too short a period to complete such an event. The achieved levels illustrate the difference in 'therapeutic' plasma concentrations between the drugs. More extensive data on analyses of those drugs in plasma following administration via various routes and in different vehicles have been published in several articles (Steffenrud, 1980; Dimov and Gréen, 1983; Gréen and Bygdeman, 1976, 1977; Bergström et al., 1976; Bygdeman et al., 1977; Gréen et al., 1978, 1982; Dimov et al., 1983). The plasma levels necessary for a uterine stimulation, strong enough for induction of abortion, are about 200–500 pg/ml for 16,16-dimethyl-PGE_2 and 16,16-dimethyl-trans-Δ^2-PGE_1; about 1.0–1.5 ng/ml for 15-methyl-$PGF_{2\alpha}$ and 15–25 ng/ml for 9-deoxo-16,16-dimethyl-9-methylene-PGE_2. Thus the introduction of the 9-

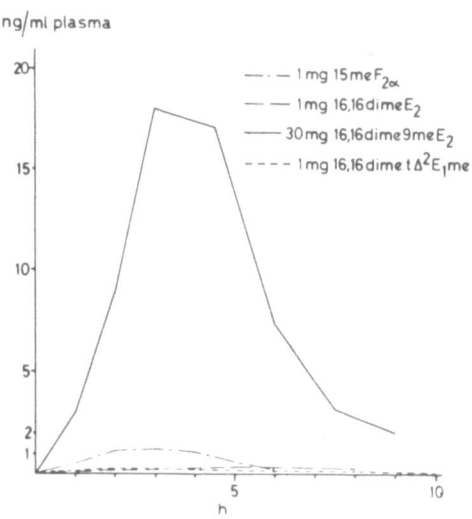

Figure 2.8 'Therapeutical' plasma levels of the four analogs

methylene instead of the 9-oxo group reduces the potency to stimulate the human uterus *in vivo* about 50 times. However, the side-effects, in terms of stimulation of gastrointestinal smooth muscle, also seem to parallell the uterotonic effect; i.e. although the plasma levels of the 9-methylene analog needed for abortion are high this does not increase the frequency of gastrointestinal side-effects.

Acknowledgements

These studies have been supported by grants from the Upjohn and the WHO Special Programme of Research, Development and Research Training in Human Reproduction.

References

Änggård, E., Larsson, C. and Samuelsson, B. (1971). The distribution of 15-hydroxy-prostaglandin dehydrogenase and prostaglandin-Δ^{13}-reductase in different tissues of the swine. *Acta Phys. Scand.*, **81**, 396

Bergström, S., Gréen, K. and Bygdeman, M. (1976). Metabolism and pharmacokinetics of 15-methyl-PGF$_{2\alpha}$ methyl ester after administration via various routes. *Prostaglandins*, Suppl. **12**, 17

Bygdeman, M., Ganguli, A., Kinoshita, K., Lundström, V., Gréen, K. and Bergström, S. (1977). Development of a vaginal suppository suitable for single administration for interruption of second trimester pregnancy. *Contraception*, **15**, 129

Dimov, V. and Gréen, K. (1983). (To be published).

Dimov, V., Gréen, K., Bygdeman, M., Konishi, Y., Imaki, K. and Hayashi, M. (1983). Gas chromatographic–mass spectrometric quantitation of 16,16-dimethyl-trans-Δ^2-PGE$_1$. *Prostaglandins* (In press)

Granström, E. and Samuelsson, B. (1969). The structure of a urinary metabolite of prostaglandin F$_{2\alpha}$ in man. *J. Am. Chem. Soc.*, **91**, 3398

Gréen, K. and Bygdeman, M. (1976). Plasma levels of the methyl ester of 15-methyl-PGF$_{2\alpha}$ in connection with intravenous and vaginal administration to the human. *Prostaglandins*, **11**, 879

Gréen, K. and Bygdeman, M. (1977). Plasma levels of 15(S)15-methyl PGF$_{2\alpha}$ following administration via various routes for induction of abortion. *Prostaglandins*, **14**, 1013

Gréen, K., Bygdeman, M. and Bremme, K. (1978). Interruption of early first trimester pregnancies by single vaginal administration of 15-methyl-PGF$_{2\alpha}$ methyl ester. *Contraception*, **18**, 551

Gréen, K., Vesterqvist, O., Bygdeman, M. and Christensen, N. J. (1982). Plasma levels of 9-deoxo-16,16-dimethyl-9-methylene-PGE$_2$ in connection with it's development as an abortifacient. *Prostaglandins*, **24**, 451

Hansson, G. and Granström, E. (1977). Metabolism of 15-methyl-prostaglandin-F$_{2\alpha}$ in the Cynomolgus monkey and the human female. *Biochem. Med.*, **18**, 420

Miller, O. V. and Magee, W. E. (1974). *In vitro* hydrolysis of prostaglandin F$_{2\alpha}$ esters by serum or plasma of different animal species. *Prostaglandins*, **7**, 29

Samuelsson, B., Granström, E., Gréen, K., Hamberg, M. and Hammarström, S. (1975). Prostaglandins. *Ann. Rev. Biochem.*, **44**, 669

Steffenrud, S. (1980). Metabolism of 16,16-dimethyl-prostaglandin E$_2$ in the human female. *Biochem. Med.*, **24**, 274

Steffenrud, S. (1983). Metabolism of 9-deoxo-16,16-dimethyl-9-methylene-PGE$_2$ in the human. *Drug Metab. Disp.*, **11**, 255

3
Prostaglandins in the regulation of non-pregnant uterine contractility

V. LUNDSTRÖM

INTRODUCTION

The identification of the primary prostaglandins PGF and PGE immediately evoked an interest in studying the effect of these prostaglandins on the myometrium. A stimulatory effect of $PGF_{2\alpha}$ and $PGF_{1\alpha}$ on uterine contractility, and in contrast a relaxing effect of PGE_2 and PGE_1 *in vitro*, was reported by Swedish investigators in the 1960s (Bygdeman, 1964; Sandberg, *et al.*, 1964, 1966). These early studies also revealed that PGE_1 and PGE_2 stimulated the proximal portion of the tube, while a relaxation was found in the distal part of the tube and the ampulla. Since then, many new prostanoids have been identified and a very complex response of the myometrium to different prostaglandins has been observed. This review will cover *in vitro* as well as *in vivo* studies on the effect of different prostaglandins on the myometrium and tube.

Recent investigators have revealed a complex response of the myometrium to prostaglandins depending on the localization of the fibers and the phase of the menstrual cycle. Therefore, the architecture of the muscle fibers within the uterus will first be identified with a step-wise dissection of the different parts. The corpus uteri is composed of three different muscle layers – namely: a thin subperitoneal layer parallel to, or in a helix along, the axis of the uterus; an intermediate irregular layer; and an internal spiral shaped layer. In the isthmic part of the uterus the muscle fibers are organized in a circular manner. Furthermore, in the uterotubal junction, three different muscle layers have been identified: an external spiral, an intermediate circular, and an internal longitudinal layer.

UTERUS *IN VITRO*

Wilhelmsson and co-workers have studied in detail the separate effects of different prostanoids on the myometrium *in vitro* (Wilhelmsson *et al.*, 1979, 1981).

PGE$_2$

Administration of PGE$_2$ inhibits the spontaneous contractility in the intermediate and the internal layer of the corpus uteri. However, the subperitoneal myometrial fibers generally react with stimulation to low doses (1 ng/ml) while higher concentrations (100 ng/ml) induce relaxation. The isthmic part of the uterus is essentially insensitive to PGE$_2$. In the uterotubal junction, PGE$_2$ induces a stimulatory response in the outer layer while the circular intermediate layer responds with relaxation. The internal longitudinal layer shows a complex response to PGE$_2$, depending on the phase of the cycle, with stimulation around ovulation and inhibition in the other phases of the cycle.

PGF$_{2\alpha}$

Addition of PGF$_{2\alpha}$ stimulates all layers of the corpus uteri. The isthmus uteri is equally insensitive to PGF$_{2\alpha}$. The uterotubal junction shows a constant stimulation to PGF$_{2\alpha}$ in all layers irrespective of the phase of the cycle. A mixture of PGF$_{2\alpha}$ and PGE$_2$ in equal concentrations causes stimulation of the corpus uteri. The ratio of PGE$_2$ to PGF$_{2\alpha}$ has to increase to 10:1 before relaxation will occur in the corpus uteri.

PGI$_2$ (prostacyclin)

Prostacyclin is synthesized within the myometrium from precursors within the endometrium. Administration of PGI$_2$ results in an inhibitory response in all muscle fibers of the myometrium irrespective of the phase of the menstrual cycle. In accordance, the muscle layers of the uterotubal junction also respond with inhibition to PGI$_2$. The efficacy of PGI$_2$ in relaxing the strips is estimated to be one-tenth of PGE$_2$.

PGH$_2$

Moderate doses of PGH$_2$ (5–100 ng/ml) elicit a stimulatory response of the myometrium. Administration of higher doses causes a biphasic response with contraction followed by subsequent relaxation. In the uterotubal layers administration of PGH$_2$ results in a stimulatory response in the muscle strips of the outer spiral and the inner layer, while inhibition is obtained in the intermediate layer.

TXA$_2$

Thromboxane is the most potent prostanoid causing stimulation of the corpus uteri as well as all layers of the uterotubal junction at very low doses (0.07 ng/ml). Thromboxane is present in the thrombocytes and it has been suggested that thromboxane in the menstrual blood may be responsible for contracting the uterotubal junction, thus avoiding retrograde menstruation.

OVIDUCT *IN VITRO*

The oviduct contains a circular and a longitudinal muscle layer. It is believed that the transport of the ovum is mediated by muscular contractions, probably elicited by prostaglandins. It is well known that the follicular fluid at ovulation contains high concentrations of prostaglandins which, after the rupture of the follicle, may act on the muscle layers within the oviduct and in the mesosalpinx. An increasing effect on the tension in the ovarian ligament may also facilitate the ovum pick-up.

The isthmus of the oviduct in the human has been extensively studied *in vitro* by Lindblom *et al.* (1978). They observed that PGE_1 and PGE_2 relax the circular muscle layer and contract the longitudinal layer. Administration of $PGF_{2\alpha}$ constantly contracts the two muscle layers in accordance with the effect on the uterus. PGI_2 has been shown to elicit a weak stimulatory response. These different responses of prostaglandins suggest an interplay on tubal function, which may mediate the opening of the isthmus under dominance of PGE_2 and locking under $PGF_{2\alpha}$ dominance.

In the ampulla, the myofibrils within the mucosal folds show a stimulatory effect of $PGF_{2\alpha}$ as expected. The effect of PGE_2 on these mucosal folds is dependent upon the phase of the cycle with increased contractility around ovulation but relaxation during all other phases. It is likely that the ratio of PGE and PGF is essential for the function of the oviduct.

IN VIVO

The contractility of the myometrium can be recorded by open-end catheter, micro-balloon, or micro-transducer. Characteristic contractility patterns are observed during the different phases of the cycle. In the proliferative phase the contractions are characterized by small amplitude of 10–30 mmHg, a frequency of 1–3 min with a resting tone of 10–25 mmHg. Around the time of ovulation the tone increases to 40–60 mmHg and the frequency increases to 3–5 min with the amplitude reduced to 5–20 mmHg. After ovulation the tone decreases to 10–30 mmHg again and the amplitude increases to 80 mmHg.

By addition of exogenous steroid hormones to menopausal women it has been shown that estrogens elicit the proliferative pattern (Bengtsson, 1966). The secretory phase pattern can similarly be evoked by the addition of gestagens. Consequently, the different patterns observed during the menstrual cycle are dependent on the steroid hormone levels. When the progesterone concentration decreases in the late secretory phase, an increased uterine activity during menstruation is recognized. Regular contractions with high amplitudes around 100–150 mmHg appear, with a basic tone around 30–50 mmHg.

Excessive endogenous synthesis of prostaglandin $F_{2\alpha}$ occurs in connection with dysmenorrhea. A uterine hypercontractility state is recorded during menstrual cramps. Administration of a potent prostaglandin biosynthesis inhibitor relaxes the myometrium within 30–60 min (Lundström *et al.*, 1976). Obviously, the synthesis of endogenous PG can rapidly be affected, thus relieving menstrual pain. The exact relationship between steroid hormones and PG synthesis is not known. It is, however, believed that PG mediates the uterine contractility following steroid hormone impulses.

THE EFFECT OF ADMINISTRATION OF PG

Intravenous administration of both PGE_2 and $PGE_{2\alpha}$ results in stimulation of the myometrium, PGE_2 generally 2–3 times more potent that $PGF_{2\alpha}$ (Roth-Brandel et al., 1970). Prostacyclin has been tested intravenously without any effect on the contractility (Wilhelmsson et al., 1981; Swahn and Lundström, 1983).

A more specific response of $PGF_{2\alpha}$ and PGE_2 is obtained when prostaglandins are injected through a thin catheter directly into the uterine cavity. Extensive studies have been performed by Martin and Bygdeman (1978). Their experiments revealed that the myometrium is most sensitive in the early proliferative and late secretory phases. During these periods, 1 μg of PGE_2 or 2–5 μg of $PGF_{2\alpha}$ elicited a strong stimulatory response. However, around ovulation the uterus was insensitive to PGE_2 and $PGF_{2\alpha}$. Doses as high as 40–50 μg may be given without effect. If the doses of PGE_2 are further increased an inhibition was found by Toppozada et al. (1974). At menstruation a complex response following PGE_2 administration is observed. Low doses of PGE_2 (2–5 μg) still stimulate the contractility while higher doses (30–40 μg) relax the myometrium. $PGF_{2\alpha}$, however, invariably stimulates uterine contractility even during menstruation.

Toppozada and co-workers reported a discrepancy between functionally infertile and normal fertile women in the uterine response to PGE_2 following local administration (Toppozada et al., 1977). A strong stimulatory response of the myometrium is observed in women with unexplained infertility at mid-cycle, while the fertile controls respond with slight inhibition. These authors indicated that an aberrant uterine response to PGE_2 at ovulation may be an etiologic factor in functional infertility.

PGI_2 injected locally into the uterine cavity elicits a gradual stimulation. This effect is probably not a direct effect of PGI_2 on the muscle fibers but rather a secondary effect of its strong vascular effect (Wilhelmsson et al., 1981; Swahn and Lundström, 1983). At this time little is known about the in vivo effect on the other prostanoids, thromboxane and endoperoxides.

CONCLUSION

The effect of the primary prostaglandins, $PGF_{2\alpha}$ and PGE_2, is studied in detail on the myometrium. Recent research has given further information on the effect of other prostanoids on the uterine activity.

References

Bengtsson, L. P. and Theobald, G. W. (1966). The effects of estrogen and gestogen on the non-pregnant human uterus. Br. J. Obstet. Gynaecol., 73, 273

Bygdeman, M. (1964). The effect of different prostaglandins on the human myometrium in vitro. *Acta Physiol. Scand.* (Suppl. 63), **242,** 1

Lindblom, B., Hamberger, L. and Wiqvist, N. (1978). Differentiated contractile effects of prostaglandin E and I on the isolated circular and longitudinal smooth muscle of the human oviduct. *Fertil. Steril.,* **30,** 533

Lindblom, B., Wikland, M. and Wiqvist, N. (1981). PGH_2, TxA_2 and PGI_2 have potent and differentiated actions on human uterine contractility. *Prostaglandins,* **21,** 277

Lundström, V., Gréen, K. and Wiqvist, N. (1976). Prostaglandins, indomethacin and dysmenorrhea. *Prostaglandins,* **11,** 893

Martin, J. N., Bygdeman, M. and Eneroth, P. (1978). The influence of locally administered prostaglandin E_2 and $F_{2\alpha}$ on uterine motility in the intact non-pregnant human uterus. *Acta Obstet. Gynecol. Scand.,* **57,** 141

Roth-Brandel, U., Bygdeman, M. and Wiqvist, N. (1970). Effects of intravenous administration of prostaglandin E, and $F_{2\alpha}$ on the contractility of the nonpregnant human uterus *in vivo. Acta Obstet. Gynecol. Scand.* (Suppl. 49), **5,** 19

Sandberg, F., Ingelman-Sundberg, A. and Rydén, G. (1964). The effect of prostaglandin E_2 and E_3 on the human uterus and Fallopian tubes in vitro. *Acta Obstet. Gynecol. Scand.,* **43,** 95

Sandberg, F., Ingelman-Sundberg, A. and Rydén, G. (1965). The effect of prostaglandin $F_{1\alpha}$, $F_{1\beta}$, $F_{2\alpha}$ and $F_{2\beta}$ on the human uterus and Fallopian tube in vitro. *Acta Obstet. Gynecol. Scand.,* **44,** 585

Swahn, M.-L. and Lundström, V. (1983). The effect of intravenous and intrauterine administration of prostacyclin on the non-pregnant uterine contractility in vivo. *Acta Obstet. Gynecol. Scand.* (Suppl. 113), **47**

Toppozada, M., Gaafar, A. and Shaala, S. (1974). *In vivo* inhibition of the human nonpregnant uterus by prostaglandin E_2. *Prostaglandins,* **8,** 401

Toppozada, M., Khowessah, M., Shaala, S., Osman, M. and Rahman, H. A. (1977). Aberrant uterine response to prostaglandin E_2 as a possible etiologic factor in functional infertility, *Fertil. Steril.,* **28,** 434

Wilhelmsson, L., Lindblom, B. and Wiqvist, N. (1979). The human uterotubal junction: contractile patterns of different smooth muscle layers and the influence of prostaglandin E_2, prostaglandin $F_{2\alpha}$ and prostaglandin I_2 in vitro. *Fertil. Steril.,* **32,** 303

Wilhelmsson, L. (1981). Biological actions of prostaglandins on different tissues within the nonpregnant human uterus. *Dissertation,* Gothenburg University, Sweden

Wilhelmsson, L., Wikland, M. and Wiqvist, N. (1981). PGH_2, TxA_2 and PGI_2 have potent and differentiated actions on human uterine contractility. *Prostaglandins,* **21,** 277

4
Effects of prostaglandins on the human non-pregnant uterus and ovary

M. K. TOPPOZADA

There are at least four fundamental areas in human reproduction where prostaglandins (PGs) are involved. These are the possible physiological role in the regulation of reproductive events, their implications in pathological situations and functional disorders, their involvement as mediators to pharmacological agents, and their application to induce therapeutic effects. Many of the suggested diverse actions and versatile roles remain conjectural due to analytical problems or difficulties in interpretation of data extracted from *in vitro* and animal experiments which may not be applicable to the human situation. Moreover, biological effects in response to pharmacological doses of PGs may not reflect a physiological role.

EFFECT OF PROSTAGLANDINS ON THE CONTRACTILITY OF THE HUMAN NON-PREGNANT UTERUS

The human non-pregnant uterus has a certain degree of spontaneous motility which varies at different phases of the menstrual cycle. The pattern of contractility is well documented but the controlling factors are not fully identified. Ovarian steroids, vasopressin and neurotransmitters, among other humoral substances, have been implicated as possible regulatory agents and the available knowledge has become even more complex and difficult to understand with the appearance of the uterotonic prostaglandins. Two main approaches attempted to reveal the involved mechanisms; either to correlate circulating or tissue levels of a humoral agent with a simultaneously recorded pattern of motility or to administer the substance of interest and evaluate the uterine response.

Studies to evaluate the uterine sensitivity or reactivity to certain drugs followed one of two main designs. The first relied on administration of small subeffective doses, gradually increasing the dose till the first recognizable response – i.e. finding the threshold dose; the lower the threshold dose the more potent the drug was and the more sensitive was the uterus to this compound. The second approach depended on administration of relatively high doses and the degree of response to a fixed dose was evaluated; the greater the response, the more sensitive was the uterus. The main parameter used to evaluate the response to PG administration was related to the degree of rise or drop in uterine tonus following drug administration (Toppozada *et al.*, 1974a, 1975; Martin *et al.*, 1978).

Uterine response to PGs in normal cycles and the menopause

Basic response to different prostaglandins

Under *in vivo* conditions, the response of the non-pregnant uterus to $PGF_{2\alpha}$ was one of stimulation at all phases of the cycle whether the compound was administered by i.v. injections or by intrauterine instillation (Shaala *et al.*, 1977). At mid-cycle (as compared to other phases) i.v. injections induced the greatest response while intrauterine instillation caused the least response (Fig. 4.1). In contrast, the response to PGE_2 was variable since a stimulation or an inhibition were elicited depending on the type of test (*in vivo* or *in vitro*), the phase of the cycle and the route of administration. Intravenous injections of PGE_2 resulted in a uterotonic response irrespective of the phase of the cycle tested (Roth-Brandel *et al.*, 1970; Coutinho and Maia, 1971; Karim *et al.*, 1971; Toppozada *et al.*, 1975). When the compound was administered locally into the uterine cavity via a thin instillation catheter the uterine response was one of stimulation in the proliferative and secretory phases but a reversal in response into one of profound inhibition was observed around ovulation time and during the first 3 days of menstruation (Toppozada *et al.*, 1975, 1977; Martin *et al.*, 1978; Toppozada *et al.*, 1980; Salem, 1982) (Figs 4.2 and 4.3).

In a series of experiments conducted in our department (Toppozada *et al.*, unpublished data) three PGE_2 metabolites (15-keto, 15-keto 13,14 dihydro and 13,14 dihydro PGE_2) were separately instilled in a dose of 500 μg into the uterine cavity at the different phases of the cycle. Relative to PGE_2, the three metabolites were less potent uterine stimulants and there were no instances of uterine inhibition. With 15-keto PGE_2, half the cases in the proliferative phase, one-third around ovulation time and all of them at the secretory phase responded by stimulation. With 15-keto, 13,14 dihydro PGE_2 all the cases reacted by stimulation at all the cycle phases. The same was observed at the proliferative and secretory phases following the instillation of 13,14 dihydro PGE_2 but around ovulation time none of the cases showed any response. The 13,14 dihydro PGE_2 metabolite was more potent than the others at the proliferative and secretory phases but the least effective around ovulation time.

One of the potent PGE_2 analogs, 16-phenoxy ω-tetranor PGE_2 methyl sulfonylamide (Sulprostone = Nalador), which is believed to be reproductive-specific, was also evaluated for its uterotonic potency at the various phases of the menstrual cycle (Toppozada *et al.*, unpublished data). The intrauterine instillation of different doses (25–200 μg) had a consistent uterine-stimulating effect in the proliferative and secretory phases while 7 out of the 18 cases tested

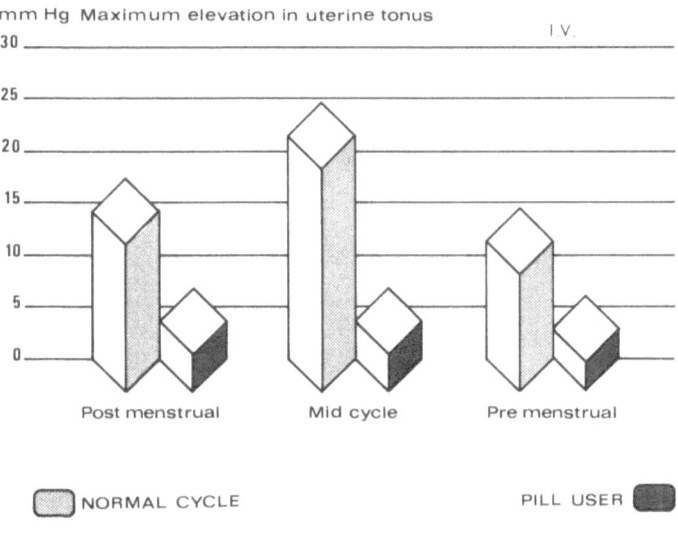

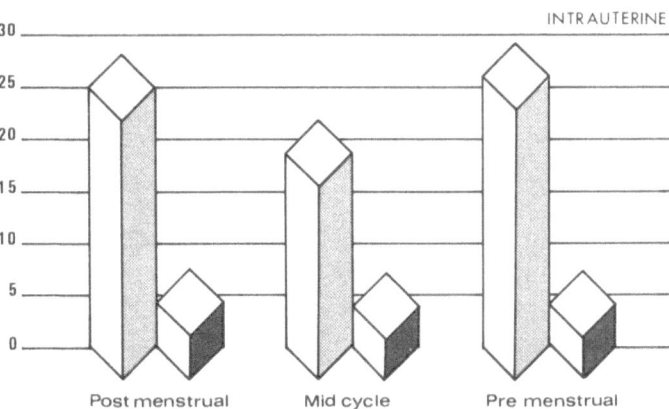

Figure 4.1 Mean of the maximum elevation in uterine tonus in response to i.v. injections (50 µg in normal and pill cycles) or intrauterine instillation (50 µg in normal cycles and 100 µg in pill users) of $PGF_{2\alpha}$. Note the markedly reduced uterine response in pill users (Shaala *et al.*, 1977)

around mid-cycle showed no response. The analog proved to be more potent than PGE_2 in this respect with a relative uterine insensitivity to its effect around ovulation time.

Studies on the uterine reactivity to PGs in the menopause showed that i. v. injections of PGE_2 or $PGF_{2\alpha}$ as well as intrauterine instillation of $PGF_{2\alpha}$ had a consistent uterine-stimulatory effect (Shaala *et al.*, 1974). However, the response was in most instances weaker than that observed in cycling women.

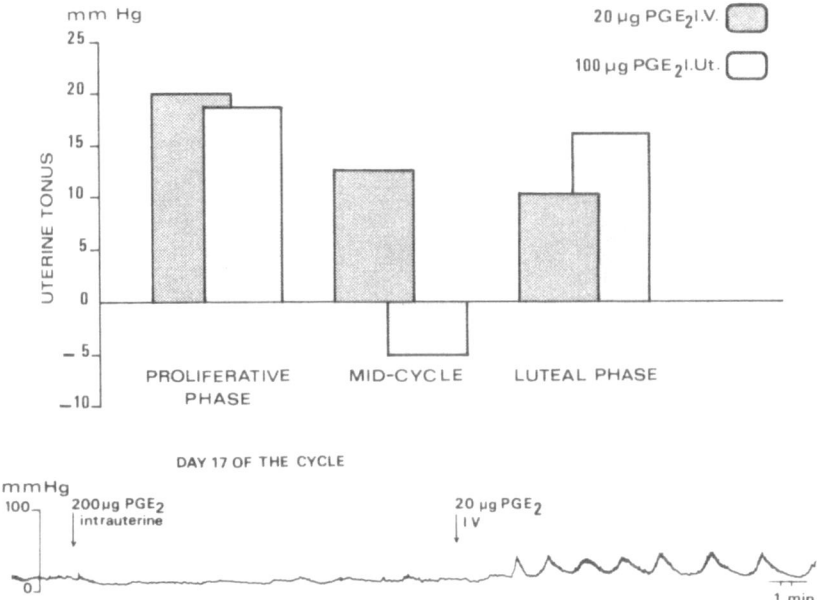

Figure 4.2 Effect of i.v. injections and intrauterine instillation of PGE$_2$ (100 µg) on the contractility of the non-pregnant human uterus in the proliferative, periovulatory and secretory phases of the menstrual cycle. Note the stimulatory effect of i.v. PGE$_2$ (20 µg) and the marked inhibition following local instillation (100 µg) around ovulation time. The upper part of the figure presents the mean values of maximum elevation or drop of tonus in response to i.v. and local PGE$_2$. The lower part shows a record of contractility on day 17 and illustrates the effect of i.v. and intrauterine PGE$_2$

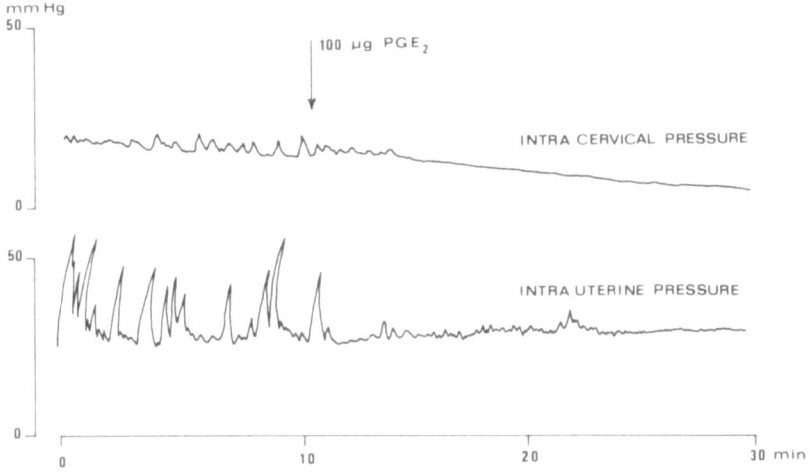

Figure 4.3 Effect of intrauterine instillation of 100 µg PGE$_2$ on uterine and cervical contractility during menstruation (day 2). Note the inhibition of uterine and cervical activity (unpublished data)

30

When PGE_2 was instilled into the uterine cavity of early menopausal women (up to 3 years) it usually caused inhibition of all contractility components, especially at the high dose range of 80–200 μg. In women who were menopausal over 3 years the uterine response to local PGE_2 was variable and inconsistent, since five cases showed a stimulatory response, one was non-reactive and four responded by inhibition. One of the latter subjects demonstrated a rebound stimulation following the phase of inhibition.

The *in-vivo* effect of PGs on the intracervical pressure in the human, though technically difficult to record, showed interesting data (Coutinho and Darzé, 1976). The i.v. injection of $PGF_{2\alpha}$ was found stimulatory to the cervix at all phases of the menstrual cycle, whereas PGE_2 was inhibitory, which was most marked during mid-cycle. The authors could not record cervical pressures during menstruation. However, our data relating to intrauterine instillation of PGE_2 during the second day of menstrual flow showed an evident uterine as well as cervical relaxation (Fig. 4.3) (Salem, 1982). After the third day of menstrual bleeding the uterine response to local PGE_2 reversed into stimulation while the cervical response remained an inhibitory one.

Thromboxane B_2, the major metabolite of thromboxane A_2, is a potent platelet aggregator and vasoconstrictor, and its role in reproductive physiology has not been adequately investigated. Thromboxane A_2 had a marked stimulatory effect on the human myometrium *in vitro*; in fact it was the most potent PG tested in this respect (Wiqvist and Wilhelmsson, 1979; Wilhelmsson, 1981). Under *in vivo* conditions the effect of local intrauterine instillation of thromboxane B_2 has recently been evaluated at the different phases of the menstrual cycle (Saleh, 1982; Toppozada *et al.*, 1983). The compound proved to be a powerful uterine stimulant at all phases of the cycle (Fig. 4.4). The greatest response was observed in the secretory phase while the least response occurred in the proliferative phase and there was no reduction in uterine sensitivity to its administration in the periovulatory phase. Its uterotonic potency during menstruation may thus be involved in the pathophysiology of primary dysmenorrhea.

Prostacyclin (PGI_2), which is a potent vasodilator and a strong inhibitor of platelet aggregation, had an inhibitory action *in vitro* on uterine smooth muscle while no significant effect on uterine contractility was noticed *in vivo* (Wilhelmsson *et al.*, 1979; Wilhelmsson, 1981; Wilhelmsson *et al.*, 1981). However, a recent study reported that i.v. infusions of PGI_2 were without effect on the contractility of the non-pregnant human uterus while local instillation of the compound induced a stimulatory response (Swahn and Lundstrom, 1983).

The major metabolite of prostacyclin, 6-keto-$PGF_{1\alpha}$, has been shown to be an *in vivo* uterine stimulant when locally instilled into the uterine cavity in relatively high doses at all phases of the cycle (Shaala *et al.*, 1983), without a single instance of inhibition (Fig. 4.5). The response (as judged by elevation in tonus and duration of response) was greatest in the secretory phase and least during menstruation.

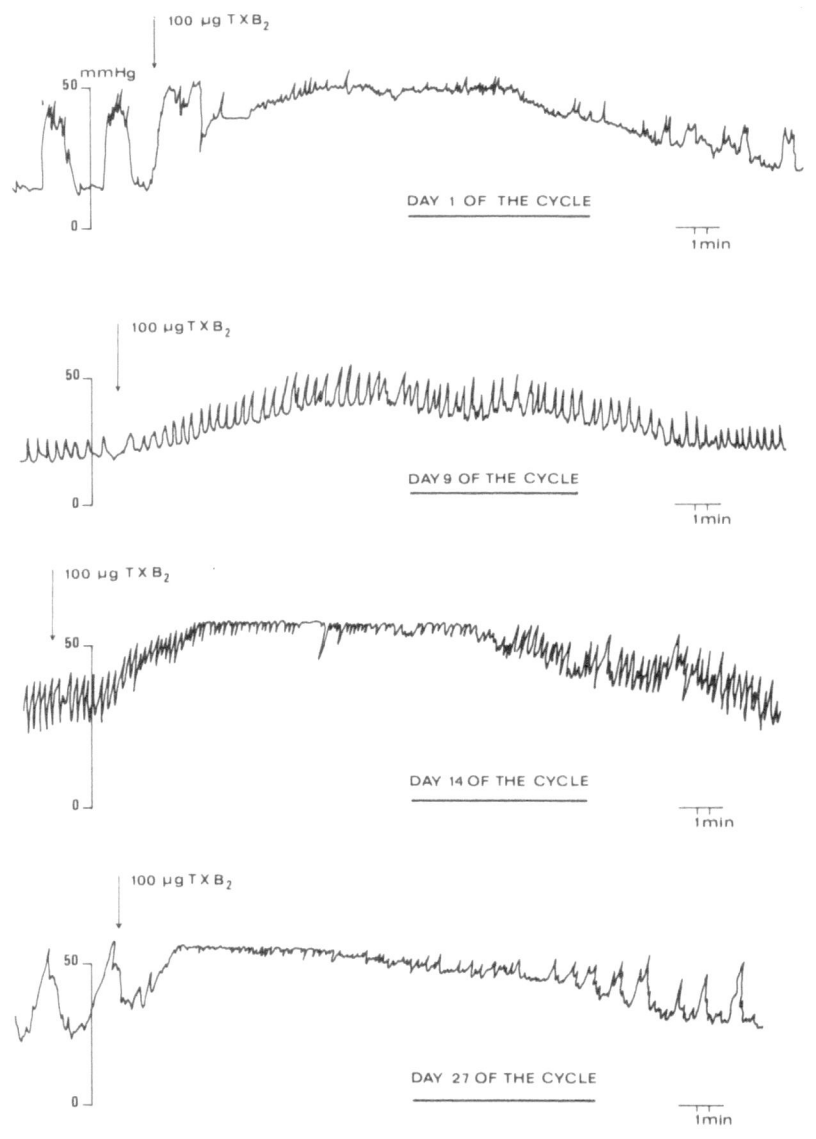

Figure 4.4 Response of the non-pregnant human uterus to intrauterine instillation of 100 μg thromboxane B_2 at the different phases of the menstrual cycle. Note the consistent powerful stimulation at all the phases (Toppozada *et al.*, 1983)

Influence of exogenous hormones on the uterine response to PG:

Estrogen–progestogen combination (oral contraceptives)

The way in which combined oral contraceptives (OC) (containing 0.05 mg ethinyl estradiol and 0.5 mg norgestrel) may modify the uterine response to

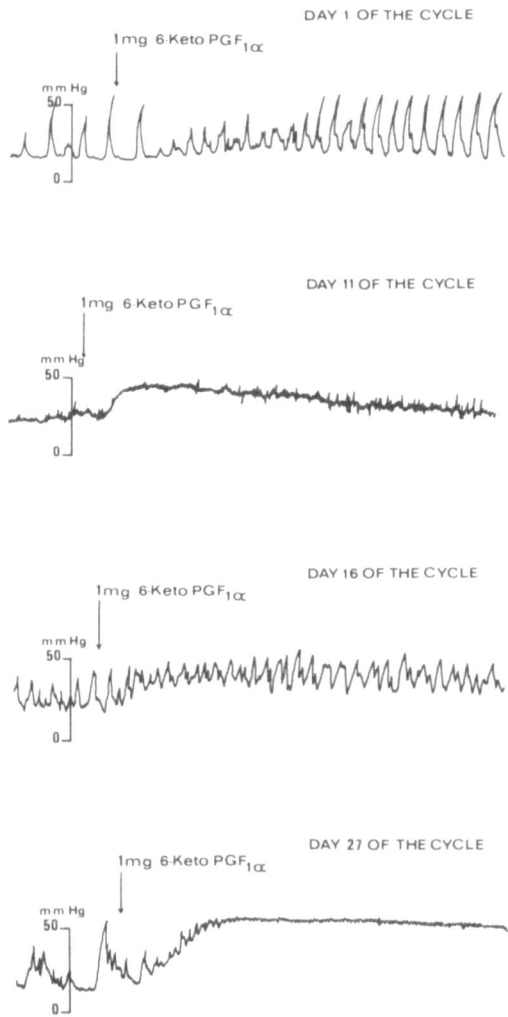

Figure 4.5 Response of the non-pregnant human uterus to local intrauterine instillation of 1 mg 6-keto-$PGF_{1\alpha}$ at the various phases of the menstrual cycle showing the consistent stimulatory effect

PG administration was evaluated in 70 fertile women (Toppozada *et al.*, 1976; Shaala *et al.*, 1977). The uterus in OC users showed a markedly reduced response to local and systemic administration of $PGF_{2\alpha}$ and to i.v. injections of PGE_2 at all phases of the cycle (Fig. 4.1). A similar suppression of reactivity was observed in the post- and pre-menstrual phases of pill users in response to local intrauterine instillation of PGE_2. At mid-cycle, however, the usual uterine inhibition following local PGE_2 in normal cycles was replaced by a consistent uterine stimulation in pill users.

These observations may explain the previously reported suppression of all contractility components due to pill intake (Csapo and Pinto-Dantas, 1966). The reduced myometrial response to PGs in pill users may also be the reason why combined OC are very effective in relieving spasmodic dysmenorrhea. Moreover, the modifications imposed upon uterine reactivity by OC, particularly the mid-cycle reversal in response to local PGE_2, may serve as an additional factor in the contraceptive mechanism of OC.

Estrogens

The effect of estrogen administration on the response of the menopausal uterus to i.v. and intrauterine administration of PGE_2 was evaluated in five volunteers. Treatment with estradiol benzoate (5 mg/day for 5 days) induced inconsistent effects on the uterine response to locally instilled PGE_2; the cases with PGE_2-induced inhibition prior to estrogen treatment showed a reversal of response into stimulation, while cases initially responding by stimulation did not reveal an evident change in response after estrogen therapy. Intravenous injections of PGE_2 induced a stimulatory response after estrogen treatment with insignificant quantitative changes (El-Dakhakhny, 1980).

Oral and injectable progestogens

The effect of progesterone treatment (i.m. 25 mg/12 h for 5 days) on the response of the menopausal uterus to PGE_2 was evaluated in five volunteers. Progesterone treatment induced qualitative and quantitative changes in the uterine response to local PGE_2. The induced stimulation prior to progesterone treatment was reversed into an inhibition after the therapy. Response to systemic administration of PGE_2 was not altered by the course of progesterone therapy (El-Dakhakhny, 1980).

The uterine response to intrauterine instillation of PGE_2 in a group of five women under minipill contraception (0.03 mg norgestrel) for more than 2 months was also investigated. The results showed that all the cases pre- and post-menstrually reacted by stimulation except one case in each phase where an initial inhibition was followed by a rebound stimulation. Around mid-cycle there was one stimulation, two reacted by inhibition and in two cases there was no response to the local administration of PGE_2. These inconsistent responses are probably a reflection of the inconsistent endocrine alterations known to occur with minipill intake, whereby ovulation is inhibited in some subjects, others may ovulate normally while some women show abnormal ovulation or deficient corpus luteum.

The long-term i.m. administration of Depot medroxyprogesterone acetate (DMPA) suppresses the basal uterine contractility in some cases while in others it resembles the type recorded in the normal secretory phase of the cycle. There was also a significant reduction in the uterine response to local intrauterine instillation of PGE_2 (El-Dakhakhny, 1980) as compared to the response in the secretory phase of normal control cycles. The least stimulatory response to PGE_2 was observed at the post-DMPA injection phase when the highest MPA levels in the circulation are known to occur.

Gonadotropins

The effect of FSH, human chorionic gonadotropin (HCG) and luteinizing hormone releasing hormone (LHRH) administration on the response of the non-pregnant uterus to PGE_2 was studied in 48 subjects in the early proliferative and mid-secretory phases of the menstrual cycle when the endogenous levels of these hormones were relatively low. The main objective for these studies was to test the hypothesis that the mid-cycle surge of gonadotropins is involved in the mid-cycle reversal in uterine response to local instillation of PGE_2.

None of the exogenously administered gonadotropins or LHRH induced any changes in the basal uterine activity patterns. The uterine response to i.v. and intrauterine PGE_2 administration after 3 days of FSH treatment was still in the form of stimulation but was reduced in most cases both in the proliferative and secretory phases of the cycle (El-Dakhakhny, 1980).

In the LHRH test group, 16 cases were studied. After recording the basal contractility pattern, PGE_2 was instilled into the uterine cavity and the response was observed until the basal pattern was regained once more. At this stage an i.v. injection of $100 \mu g$ LHRH was given, and any effect on uterine activity was noticed for 20–30 min, then the same dose of intrauterine PGE_2 was administered again to evaluate whether the LHRH (or its induced LH peak) had any influence on the response. The induced LH peak after LHRH was confirmed in all the studied cases. It should be emphasized that in this investigation the same subject was tested twice for the response to intrauterine administration of the same dose of PGE_2 in the same session of recording; once before and once after LHRH injection, i.e. under the same humoral, nervous and psychic conditions.

Before the LHRH injection, PGE_2 instillation induced an elevation in uterine tonus in all the cases. Twenty to thirty minutes after the LHRH injection, the same dose of intrauterine PGE_2 did not induce any response in three cases, one case responded by stimulation and 12 cases reacted by marked uterine inhibition (Fig. 4.6) (El-Tarahony, 1982).

In another group of 12 cases, the response to local PGE_2 was evaluated twice, separated by an interval of 2 days where HCG was administered (1500 IU every 8 h). Before HCG, the uterus responded to local PGE_2 by stimulation in all the cases, while after the 2 days of HCG treatment the intrauterine instillation of the same dose of PGE_2 induced no response in five cases. Uterine stimulation occurred in four cases and an inhibitory response was recorded in three cases (Fig. 4.7).

Thus, both LHRH and HCG could significantly modify the uterine response to local administration of PGE_2 both qualitatively and quantitatively. Since LHRH has a half-life of about 4 min, then the changes in uterine response to local PGE_2 that was administered 20–30 min after LHRH injection were not due to the LHRH but probably due to the effect of the released LH or FSH.

The presented data incriminate LH, and to a lesser extent FSH, in the mechanism of the altered uterine reactivity to PGs around mid-cycle. Moreover, the uterine inhibition following local instillation of PGE_2 in the first 3 days of menstruation, though difficult to explain on the basis of these

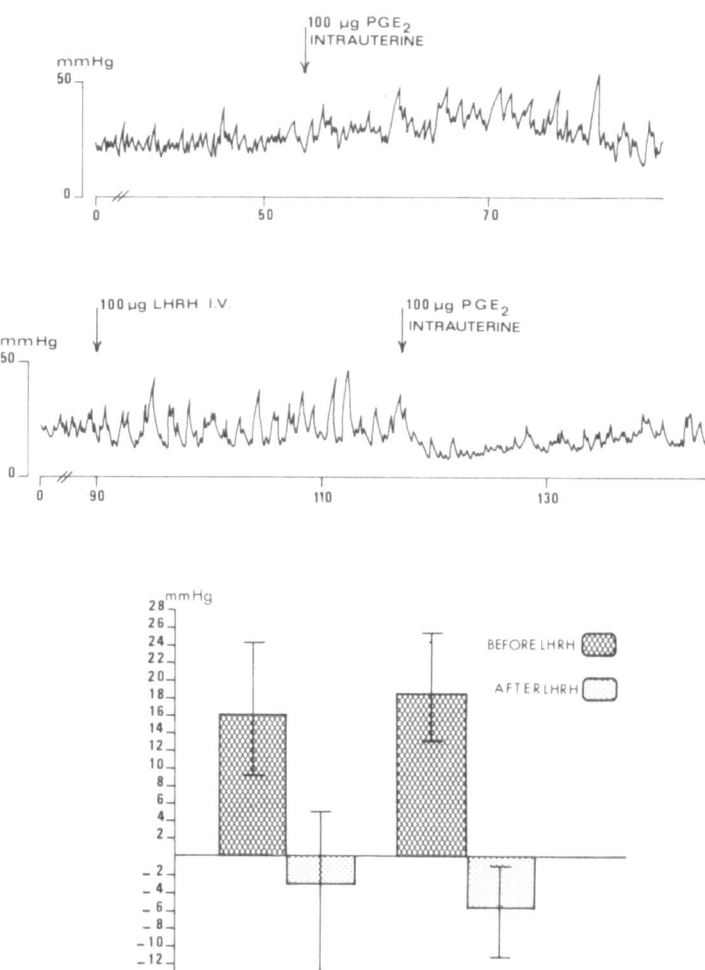

Figure 4.6 Uterine response following intrauterine instillation of PGE_2 at the secretory phase of the cycle before and after LHRH injection. Note the reversal in response to PGE_2 from stimulation before LHRH to obvious inhibition after the LHRH administration. Lower part of the figure shows the mean of the maximum elevation or drop in tonus in response to local PGE_2 before and after i.v. LHRH in the proliferative and secretory phases

data, may be related to the normal premenstrual rise in FSH. These results may also explain some of the perplexing data on the uterine response to PGs in the menopause; the uterine inhibition following local PGE_2 in the early menopause may be related to the high level of gonadotropins in this phase of life, while the observed instances of uterine stimulation in late menopausal cases may have been due to the declining levels of gonadotropins.

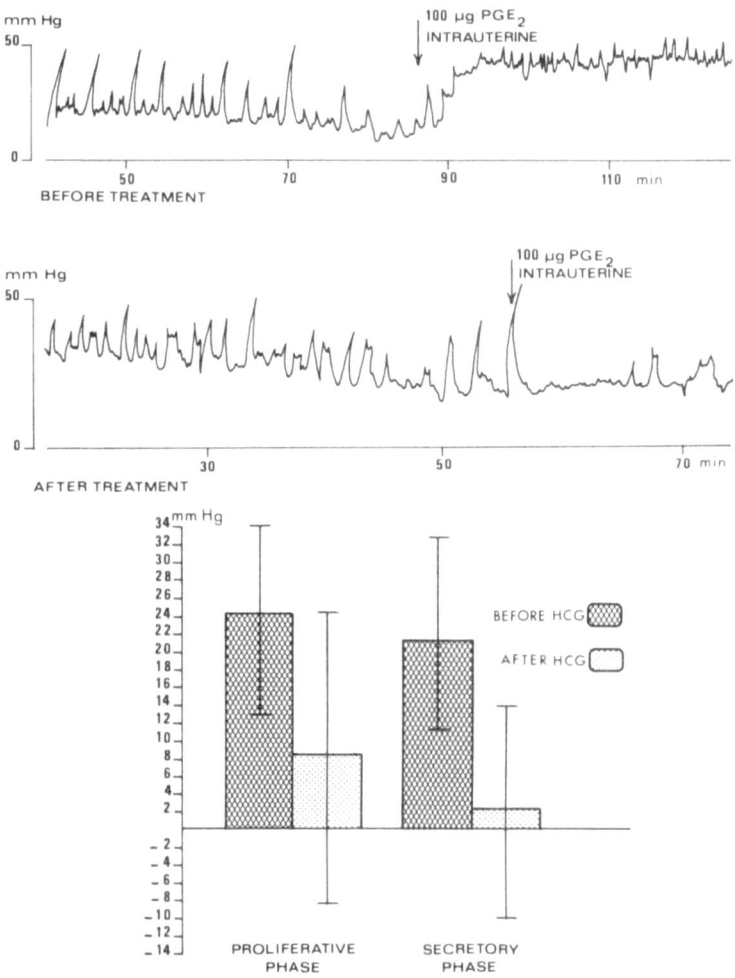

Figure 4.7 Effect of HCG treatment for 2 days on the response of the non-pregnant uterus (in the secretory phase) to intrauterine instillation of PGE_2. Note the stimulation before and inhibition after HCG therapy. The lower part of the figure shows the mean of the maximum elevation or drop in tonus.

The mechanism by which LH (and possibly FSH also) may alter the *in vivo* myometrial sensitivity to local PGE_2 is hard to explain at the present time since many complex interrelated factors may be involved, such as receptor levels, metabolic alterations and other humoral agents. Moreover, LH can produce alterations in the circulating levels of ovarian steroids (mainly estrogens) a few minutes after injection, which in turn may be implicated in the observed changes.

The results of the study with HCG were rather similar to that of LHRH but the suppression of reactivity to PGE_2 after HCG administration was less. Since HCG is secreted in large amounts during pregnancy, one would expect that the pregnant uterus would either not respond, or would react by inhibition following local instillation of PGE_2. However, it is well established that intrauterine instillation of PGE_2 during pregnancy results in a powerful stimulation. This does not of necessity contradict the presented data in the non-pregnant state, since the humoral situation during pregnancy is totally different from that normally present in non-pregnant women.

Influence of IUDs on the uterine response to PGs

The uterine activity was recorded at the different phases of the menstrual cycle (menstrual, proliferative, periovulatory and secretory) in 10 healthy non-pregnant women during a control cycle and in a cycle following IUD insertion (Lippe's Loop size C) (Toppozada et al., 1980). The presence of the IUD in the uterus increased the spontaneous uterine contractility in three cases in the proliferative phase in seven cases around ovulation time, in eight cases in the luteal phase and in all the cases during menstruation. This tendency towards hypermotility due to IUDs may contribute to abnormal bleeding and cramps that sometimes occur with IUDs. The increased and modified uterine activity after IUD insertion may also be involved, at least in part, in the IUD mechanism of action.

Following IUD insertion there was an increased uterine sensitivity to local intrauterine instillation of PGE_2 at the proliferative and luteal phases (Fig. 4.8). The uterine response around ovulation time was totally reversed after IUD insertion in the sense that stimulation resulted instead of the usual inhibition observed in control cycles (Fig. 4.8). The increased or altered uterine reactivity to PGs as a result of IUD insertion may explain the observed post-insertional changes in basal motility which may be a response to endogenously released PGs irrespective of the controversial issue whether PG release is increased or not by IUDs. Moreover, the reversed mid-cycle uterine response to local PGE_2 may add a new dimension to the mechanism of action of IUDs (Toppozada and Hafez, 1979; Toppozada et al., 1980).

Uterine response to PGs in some functional disorders:

Functional infertility

The entity of functional infertility is well known and still remains unexplained and lacking a proper line of management. Among many hypothetical assumptions, low levels of seminal PGE compounds (Bygdeman et al., 1970), a deficient seminal hydroxy PG derivative (Svanborg et al., 1982) and abnormal behavior in uterine motility were introduced as possible factors in the etiology of this condition.

The uterine response to PGE_2 and $F_{2\alpha}$ administration (i.v. and intra-uterine) was evaluated during the different phases of the menstrual cycle in 20 normal controls and in five functionally infertile women. The latter cases were carefully selected following exhaustive investigations of all possible factors

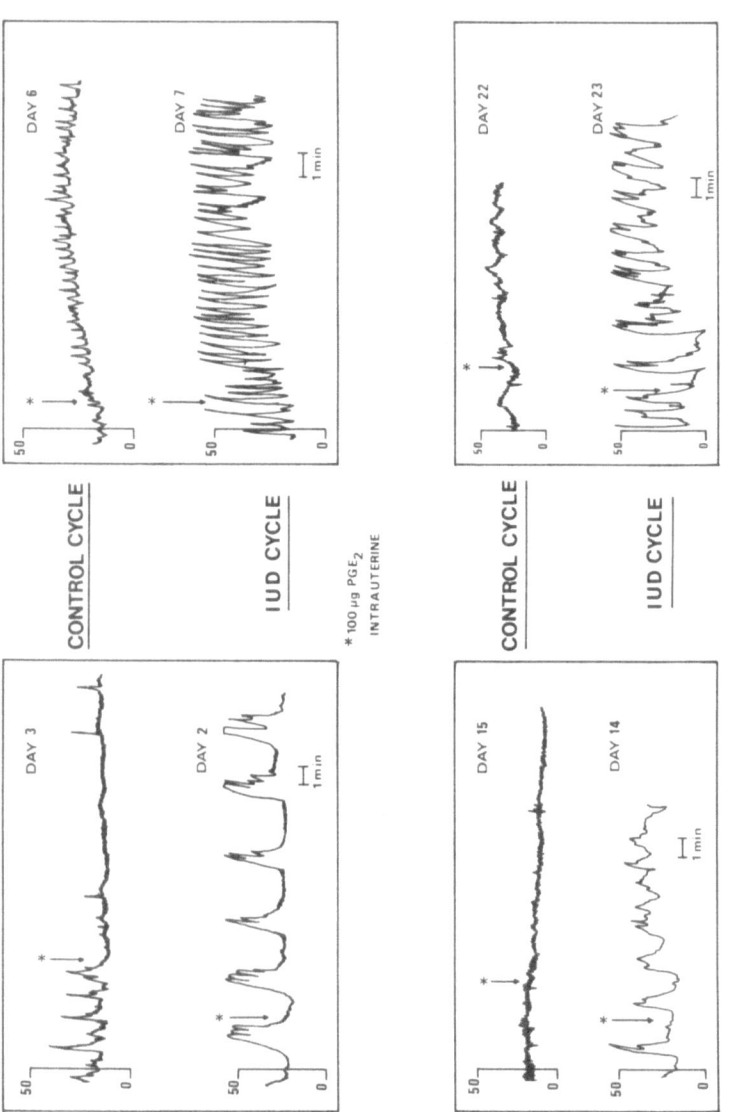

Figure 4.8 Response of the non-pregnant uterus to local instillation of PGE_2 at the different phases of a control menstrual cycle and in a cycle after IUD insertion in the same subjects

including laparoscopy, endocrine and immunologic studies. There were no apparent differences between the two groups with respect to the uterine response to either compound (systemic or local) when given in the proliferative or luteal phases of the cycle. However, at mid-cycle around ovulation time there was a marked deviation in the type of response following local instillation of PGE_2; in the normal fertile group there was definite inhibition of uterine motility, while uteri of functionally infertile women showed marked stimulation (Toppozada et al., 1977) (Fig. 4.9). The possible role of this aberrant uterine response in the etiology of functional infertility has thus been added to the existing list of causes. However, the reason for such an aberrant uterine response in functionally infertile women is unclear, and methods to rectify it are lacking.

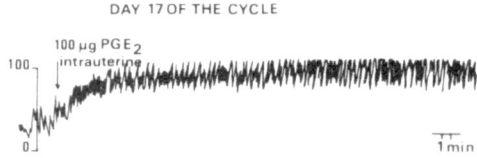

DAY 17 OF THE CYCLE

Figure 4.9 Uterine response to intrauterine instillation of PGE_2 in a functionally infertile subject at mid-cycle. Note the marked stimulation instead of the expected inhibition in normal women at this phase of the cycle.

Spasmodic dysmenorrhea

The long list of factors which may contribute to the pathophysiology of dysmenorrhea includes the presence of a uterotonic substance in the menstrual fluid. Reference to such a mysterious agent dates back to the early twenties of this century and the name 'menotoxin' was suggested (Schick, 1920). Several decades later a series of investigations revealed the nature of this material as a complex mixture of acidic and non-acidic compounds that were collectively named 'the menstrual stimulant' (Clithero and Pickles, 1961). The unidentified substance has been crudely extracted and found to cause powerful myometrial stimulation and induce changes in the tone of endometrial blood vessels and thus was implicated in the mechanism of dysmenorrhea and initiation of menstruation (Pickles, 1959). It is by now almost clear that the active principles in the menstrual fluid dealt with in past studies are a group of PGs that also exist in the endometrium (Clithero and Pickles, 1961; Pickles et al., 1965; Lundstrom and Green, 1978; Maathuis and Kelly, 1978).

Based upon a large number of publications, there seems to be a general consensus that PGs are somehow involved in the pathogenesis of dysmenorrhea. A triad of evidence in support of this theory now exists:

(1)   The level of PGs in the plasma, endometrium, menstrual discharge, and endometrial jet wash specimens of dysmenorrheic women is significantly greater as compared to non-symptomatic subjects (Halbert et al., 1975; Lundstrom and Green, 1978).

(2)   The identified raised PGs are capable of inducing spastic myometrial contractions *in vivo* similar to those observed in association with dysmenorrhea.

(3)   PG synthesis inhibitors reduce PG levels with simultaneous suppression of contractions and control of dysmenorrheic pain.

Thus a role for PGs in causing menstrual pain may appear at first glance to be clear-cut, but the situation is far from being resolved. So many complex issues and interacting factors have not been identified, and many questions remain to be answered. Is it the PGF/PGE ratio in the menstrual discharge that counts? What is the role of PGI_2, the thromboxanes and other arachidonic acid derivatives in this respect? What is the role of PG receptors? and what generates the excessive production of PGs in dysmenorrheic cases? what is the interaction between PGs and other uterotonic and vasoactive substances as well as neurotransmitters? Does a spastic cervix contribute to the induced pain? Is abnormal or increased myometrial sensitivity to certain PGs involved in the mechanism or not? Is there a deficiency of PG dehydrogenase enzyme system? Is there an increased uterine vascular sensitivity to PGs or PG-induced sensitization of uterine nerve endings?

In spasmodic dysmenorrhea there is excessive and abnormal uterine activity; the amplitude of contractions is increased, the tonus is elevated and frequently there are complex waves with no relaxation in between individual contractions (Filler and Warner, 1970; Lundstrom *et al.*, 1976). Moreover, deficient uterine polarity with hypertonic isthmus has also been observed in subjects with primary dysmenorrhea (Mann *et al.*, 1962). Uterine hyper-contractility leads to ischemia, which is believed to be a major factor in causing the dysmenorrheic pain. During each contraction local endometrial blood flow decreased simultaneously with perception of maximum colicky pain (Akerlund *et al.*, 1976). The ischemia seems to be caused primarily by mechanical compression induced by hypercontractility, but other factors acting directly on uterine vasculature may also contribute to the decreased blood flow (Akerlund *et al.*, 1976; Akerlund, 1979). Apart from uterine ischemia, PGs can also sensitize pain receptors and nerve endings. Moreover, extragenital manifestations of the dysmenorrhea syndrome – such as diar-rhea, vomiting, headache and syncope – can be produced by i.v. injections of PGs (Rosenwaks and Jones, 1980).

Plasma levels of $PGF_{2\alpha}$ and its metabolites (Lundstrom and Green, 1978) were significantly higher in dysmenorrheic women, and treatment with oral contraceptives or naproxen induced a considerable decrease in the levels of these compounds among dysmenorrheic subjects with concomitant pain relief (Lundstrom and Green, 1978; Pulkkinen *et al.*, 1978). At the local level, the concentrations of PGs of the F series were also increased in the endometrium, menstrual fluid and jet wash specimens among cases with painful menstru-ation (Pickles *et al.*, 1965; Halbert *et al.*, 1975; Lundstrom and Green, 1978).

Infusions of $PGF_{2\alpha}$ resulted in typical menstrual pain and also induced hypercontractility compatible with the pattern observed during phases of dysmenorrhea (Roth-Brandel *et al.*, 1970). The uterus was highly sensitive to the stimulatory effect of $PGF_{2\alpha}$ during painful menstruation but the uterine response was rather similar to that achieved in normal women, i.e. the dysmenorrheic uterus was not more sensitive to $PGF_{2\alpha}$ (Lundstrom, 1977; Bygdeman et al., 1979; Salem, 1982). PGE_2, on the other hand, was inhibitory during menstruation both in normal and dysmenorrheic subjects. These findings support the original hypothesis of Pickles et al., in that a high $PGF_{2\alpha}/PGE_2$ ratio may be the crucial factor in the causation of dysmenorrhea (Pickles et al., 1965). The role of the cervix in this connection has recently been evaluated, revealing that during menstruation PGE_2 inhibits cervical activity while $PGF_{2\alpha}$ and indomethacin had no effect in this respect both in dysmenorrheic and non-dysmenorrheic subjects (Salem, 1982).

Systemic administration of non-steroidal anti-inflammatory drugs, (NSAID), which inhibit PG synthesis, suppressed uterine contractility in normal and dysmenorrheic women (Lundstrom et al., 1976; Pulkkinen, 1979). Local intrauterine instillation of mefenamic acid also suppressed uterine activity, probably after its initial systemic absorption rather than by a direct effect on the myometrium since the onset of response took a similar time or even longer to appear as compared to rectal or oral administration (Salem, 1982). Intravenous infusion of $PGF_{2\alpha}$ at a low rate of 18 μg/min in a dysmenorrheic volunteer already treated with indomethacin caused a return of hypermotility and severe cramps, indicating that the NSAID did not interfere with the action of exogenous $PGF_{2\alpha}$ (Lundstrom et al., 1979).

EFFECT OF PROSTAGLANDINS ON THE HUMAN OVARY

A large number of publications showed that PGs play an important role in the regulation of various functions of the ovary. Most of the available evidence accumulated from animal data, while human investigations were few due to obvious limitations. This section will deal mainly with the human, and to a lesser extent the monkey and the subprimate ovary.

Steroidogenesis and luteolysis

The classical PGs, especially PGE_2, increased the in vitro production of progesterone and 20α progesterone by human corpora lutea obtained from the luteal phase of the menstrual cycle (Patwardhan and Lanthier, 1974; Marsh and Lemaire, 1974). Also, PGE_2 stimulated the in vitro utilization of progesterone to form 17-OH progesterone, androstenedione and 17-β estradiol in corpus luteum tissue (Marsh and Lemaire, 1974). LH was more potent than PGs as a luteal stimulant, and both PGE_2 and LH stimulated cyclic AMP in the test system; but whether their effect is additive or whether PG potentiates or mediates the gonadotropic response has not been fully resolved. When both LH and PGE_2 were added together the LH effect was inhibited, thus the luteotropic effect of PGs in vitro was reversed to a luteolytic response when combined with LH (Channing, 1972).

The effect of $PGF_{2\alpha}$ on corpora lutea in vitro is more complex and controversial than that of PGE_2. Some studies reported $PGF_{2\alpha}$ to be a weaker stimulant of luteal progesterone synthesis *in vitro* while other investigations demonstrated the inhibitory effect of $PGF_{2\alpha}$ in this respect. The discrepancies were explained on the basis of the type of test system used (corpus luteum slices, luteal cells or organ culture), the dose, the stage of luteal development, or as a biphasic response with initial stimulation followed by a luteolytic effect.

The human corpus luteum has specific receptors for PG binding. Two classes of $PGF_{2\alpha}$ receptors have been identified, one with high affinity and the other with low affinity (Powell *et al.*, 1974). The mere binding of $PGF_{2\alpha}$ to its receptor in the luteal cell membrane does not consistently induce a luteolytic response, and other concomitant humoral changes may be necessary such as changes in ovarian steroids, norepinephrine or oxytocin.

Physiological luteolysis

What controls the life span of the human corpus luteum is still unknown. It may result from withdrawal of a luteotropic agent, appearance of a luteolytic factor or release of a substance that blocks the effect of a luteotropic stimulus at the ovarian level. $PGF_{2\alpha}$ appeared to fit rather well as a luteolytic substance or a factor interfering with luteotropic stimulation. A series of elegant experiments involving several years of hard work revealed that $PGF_{2\alpha}$ (and possibly other arachidonic acid derivatives) is probably the uterine factor, formerly termed 'uterine luteolysin', which is responsible for the physiological regression of luteal function in subprimate animals (McCracken, 1971; Green *et al.*, 1972). At the time in the estrus cycle when the corpus luteum undergoes spontaneous normal regression, the uterus releases $PGF_{2\alpha}$. The physiological stimulus for $PGF_{2\alpha}$ release at that exact time is not definitely identified in all species but a role for estradiol, progesterone and oxytocin has been suggested (Poyser, 1981). The manner by which this uterine luteolysin gains access to the nearby ovary has also been investigated, showing that the anatomical vascular intimate relations between the uterine vein and ovarian artery allow the released uterine $PGF_{2\alpha}$ to cross by a countercurrent mechanism from the vein (where $PGF_{2\alpha}$ concentrations are high) to the artery, thus providing high levels to the ovary (McCracken, 1971).

When this theory was extrapolated to the primate situation many problems appeared, indicating that the primate uterus does not control corpus luteum function, and $PGF_{2\alpha}$ *per se* may not be the physiological luteolytic factor. The lack of uterine control upon the corpus luteum in humans is supported by several studies showing that hysterectomy or congenital absence of the uterus do not alter the life span of the corpus luteum (Doyle *et al.*, 1971; Coyotupa *et al.*, 1973). Moreover, it was repeatedly stated that the utero-ovarian vascular connections and mechanisms regulating ovarian function in primates are significantly different from those in subprimates. However, this assumption has been disputed in the human by showing that the vascular anatomy of the sheep was very similar to that of the human where spiral arteries were also found to run in close contact, or even within the venous walls of the mesovarian region (Bendz, 1977). This work has also shown that a countercurrent system of transfer may also exist in humans. The physiological significance of these findings is yet unidentified, but may serve the purpose of a local humoral transfer (e.g. PGs or steroids) across the vessel walls, thus creating local arterial concentrations exceeding those of the systemic arterial blood.

The other question which deserves consideration is related to whether or not $PGF_{2\alpha}$ (from sources other than the uterus) is the luteolytic factor in humans. The available data in this connection are still controversial. The presence of specific receptors for $PGF_{2\alpha}$ in the human luteal cell wall points towards some physiologic role (Powell et al., 1974). On the other hand, most studies involving exogenous administration of PGs to humans revealed absence of luteolysis. However, few investigations reported either a transient or a sustained luteolytic response (see below).

It has been suggested that PGs may be locally formed in the ovary, and these induce luteolysis (Plunkett et al., 1975), i.e. the ovary may control its own function as a type of autoregulation. The site of this PG production may be the corpus luteum itself, or may be from other ovarian compartments then carried by countercurrent transfer mechanisms to the arteriole feeding the corpus luteum. To verify these assumptions, several studies attempted to measure the concentration of $PGF_{2\alpha}$ in human corpora lutea with conflicting results; two studies reported an increase in $PGF_{2\alpha}$ in the luteal phase, one reported a drop in levels while one investigation showed that the $PGF_{2\alpha}$ levels remained unchanged (Challis et al., 1976; Shutt et al., 1976; Swanston et al., 1977; Patwardhan and Lanthier, 1981). Apart from the absolute increase in luteal $PGF_{2\alpha}$ synthesis, some authors reported an increase in the PGF/PGE ratio in the late corpus luteum of humans and monkeys as an important factor that modifies the balance towards induction of physiological luteolysis (Patwardhan and Lanthier, 1981).

Different theories attempted to explain the mechanism of the luteolytic effect of $PGF_{2\alpha}$. The vascular theory was based on constriction of the utero-ovarian vein, thus reducing ovarian flow leading to anoxia. This hypothesis was later disputed and another vascular daughter theory was introduced implicating $PGF_{2\alpha}$ in inducing vascular redistribution within the ovary with selective reduction in the blood flow to the corpus luteum. The second theory is the biochemical theory, which suggests that $PGF_{2\alpha}$ is capable of exerting a powerful direct effect on the luteal cell, thereby directly inhibiting steroidogenesis.

The stimulatory effect of LH is mediated via activation of adenylate cyclase system in the luteal cell membrane to produce the 'second messenger' cyclic adenosine monophosphate (cAMP). The cAMP-dependent protein kinases are capable of phosphorylating the luteal cell cholesterol esterase to produce an active form which will then convert the cholesterol ester into free cholesterol that is readily metabolized to progesterone (Henderson and McNatty, 1975).

It has been suggested that $PGF_{2\alpha}$ acts by blocking the stimulus required to activate adenylate cyclase by LH without interfering with its activation by other hormones having a separate specific unit (Henderson and McNatty, 1975). An additional effect on LH receptors could not be ruled out. The preovulatory surge of LH saturates the regulatory units of luteal cell which protects the corpus luteum. The dissociation of LH from its receptor is a slow process taking several days and makes the corpus luteum increasingly susceptible to the luteolytic action of $PGF_{2\alpha}$ through promoting plasma membrane $PGF_{2\alpha}$ uptake. Moreover, under the influence of progesterone there is probably an increased secretion of ovarian $PGF_{2\alpha}$. Thus with progressive aging of the corpus luteum there is more $PGF_{2\alpha}$ production and facilitated uptake by the plasma membrane which blocks the activation of adenylate cyclase and inhibits progesterone synthesis. The reason for the antagonistic effect of $PGF_{2\alpha}$ on HCG or LH actions in the aging corpus luteum, and not the younger one, was postulated to result from the dramatic increase in the corpus luteum content of noradrenaline around 5–7 days after ovulation (Hamberger et al., 1979, 1980).

The role of prostacyclin in the regulation of human ovarian steroidogenesis has not been fully explored. It was reported that prostacyclin is the predominant product from prostaglandin endoperoxide metabolism in the uterus and corpus luteum (Sun et al., 1977). Moreover, in human ovarian follicles the main prostaglandin fraction was 6-keto-$PGF_{1\alpha}$ and PGE_2 amounts were insignificant, while in the fully developed corpus luteum the ratio was reversed (Liedtke and Seifert, 1978). The effect of prostacyclin on the spontaneous contractile activity of isolated human ovarian veins was studied showing that PGI_2 depressed the tone at low concentrations and induced tone stimulation accompanied by phasic contractions with higher doses (Borda et al., 1979). These data made the authors speculate that in women under estrogenic dominance PGI_2 may be important for the regulation of the venous flow, and can play a pumping role in the countercurrent mechanism between veins and arteries in the ovarian pedicle.

Several other studies reported data opposing the theory of a physiological PG role as a luteolytic factor in humans where administration of PG synthetase inhibitors appeared not to prolong the life span of the corpus luteum (Chaudhuri and Elder, 1976; Toppozada et al., 1978, 1979).

Pathological (abnormal functional) luteolysis

Some ovarian luteal dysfunctions of unknown cause may, in theory, result from abnormal rate of PG production. Thus, if $PGF_{2\alpha}$ serves as a luteolytic agent in the human, then excessive production of this compound may lead to the syndrome of corpus luteum deficiency or insufficiency and its short life span. Recently an increase in $PGF_{2\alpha}$ has been reported in these cases (Itoh and Kunimoto, 1981). On the other hand, a prolonged life span of the corpus luteum (persistent corpus luteum) may also result from a deficiency in PG production, but this hypothesis has not been tested so far in humans.

Pharmacological luteolysis

Systemic administration of high doses of $PGF_{2\alpha}$ to the monkey inhibited corpus luteum function, as evidenced by a significant drop in progesterone secretion (Kirton, 1975). However, the systemic administration of $PGF_{2\alpha}$ to the human female did not induce a definite and sustained luteolytic response. This controversy between the human and subhuman primate was explained on the basis of a difference in the administered dose; we can give doses to the monkey that can by no means be administered safely to the human. The relatively small amounts given to the human female are further inactivated in the lungs prior to reaching the ovaries. Accordingly, what gains access to ovarian tissues represent only trace concentrations that are pharmacologically ineffective.

A large number of publications evaluated the luteolytic effects of different PGs in a wide range of designs using various routes of administration in the early, mid or late parts of the luteal phase of the human female (Table 4.1). The wide spectrum of methodology applied in these investigations also resulted in diverse and conflicting conclusions regarding the therapeutic induction of human luteolysis. In most studies, i.v. or vaginal administration of $PGF_{2\alpha}$, PGE_2, 16-phenoxy PGE_2 or 17-phenyl $PGF_{2\alpha}$ did not alter luteal function, or only induced a transient fall in progesterone secretion followed by spontaneous recovery of steroidogenesis (Wiqvist et al., 1971; Hillier et al., 1972; Jewelewicz et al., 1972; Tom et al., 1972; Lehmann et al., 1972; Lemaire and Shapiro, 1972; Jones and Wentz, 1972; Wentz and Jones, 1972, 1973; Bolognese and Corson, 1973; Henzl et al., 1973; Coudert et al., 1974; Okamura et al., 1974; Leader et al., 1976; Abdalla et al., 1979; Rahman et al., 1982). The 15-methyl analog of $PGF_{2\alpha}$, being more potent than the parent PG and having a high affinity for the luteal $PGF_{2\alpha}$ receptors, could induce a sustained luteolytic response in 8 out of 10 volunteers (Toppozada et al., 1972; Powell et al., 1974; Toppozada et al., 1981) (Fig. 4.10). The administered infusions did not alter estradiol levels, which indicates a specific effect only on luteal progesterone synthesis or that the interference with estradiol production may require a higher dose.

Vaginal administrations of a single long-acting suppository of 15-methyl $PGF_{2\alpha}$ (2.5–3 mg) at the expected time of menses in non-pregnant women did not alter the progesterone or estradiol levels; the treatment only induced vaginal spotting and menses occurred at the expected time, i.e. the therapy was not luteolytic (Kinoshita et al., 1979).

Intrauterine administration of $PGF_{2\alpha}$ in a dose of 500–2000 μg and repeated at 2-hourly intervals on six occasions induced no luteolytic effects in any of the subjects treated in the early, mid, or late luteal phases of the menstrual cycle (Lyneham et al., 1975). On the other hand, a clear luteolytic effect of $PGF_{2\alpha}$ given by the intrauterine route in physiological doses was reported in monkeys (Einer-Jensen, 1973). Several 15-methyl $PGF_{2\alpha}$ analogs or $PGF_{2\alpha}$, 1-15 lactone were tested for their luteolytic effects in the non-pregnant rhesus monkey during concomitant stimulation of the corpus luteum with HCG. A clear luteolytic response could be demonstrated following i.m. administration of many of these analogs. Other $PGF_{2\alpha}$ analogs (ICI 80996 and 81008) were also shown to be powerful luteolytic agents when given subcutaneously or per vaginum to pigtail monkeys (Russell, 1975).

Delivery of PG compounds ($F_{2\alpha}$ or 15-methyl $F_{2\alpha}$) directly to the ovary by intra-luteal injections resulted in profound luteolysis but saline injections also induced a similar effect (Toppozada et al., 1974b; Korda et al., 1975; Toppozada, 1975). These data do not confirm the luteolytic property of PGs in humans, but also do not rule out such potential. The ability of PGs to

Table 4.1 The effect of different PGs given by various routes of administration on the human luteal function (summary of different studies)

Route	PG	Duration (hours)	Dose	Luteolytic effect
Intravenous	$F_{2\alpha}$	3.5–14	4.0–250 µg/min	Absent, slight or transient
	15-me-PGF$_{2\alpha}$	6.0–16.0	0.5–7.2 µg/min	Transient or sustained
	E$_2$	6.0–8.0	4.5–15.0 µg/min	Absent or transient
	16-phenoxy-PGE$_2$	3.0	4.2 µg/min	Absent
	17-phenyl-PGF$_{2\alpha}$	16	0.4–12.0 µg/min	Transient
Vaginal	$F_{2\alpha}$	2–48	25–400 mg	Absent or transient
	15-me-PGF$_{2\alpha}$ me-ester	24	2.5–4.0 mg	Absent
Intrauterine	$F_{2\alpha}$	12	3–12 mg	Absent
Intra-luteal	$F_{2\alpha}$	—	0.5–1.0 mg	Sustained

47

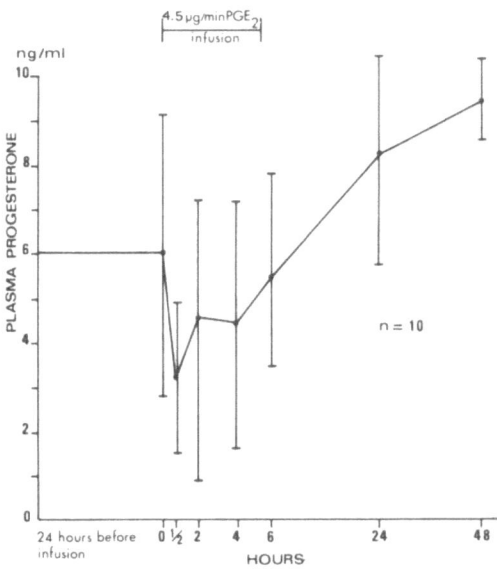

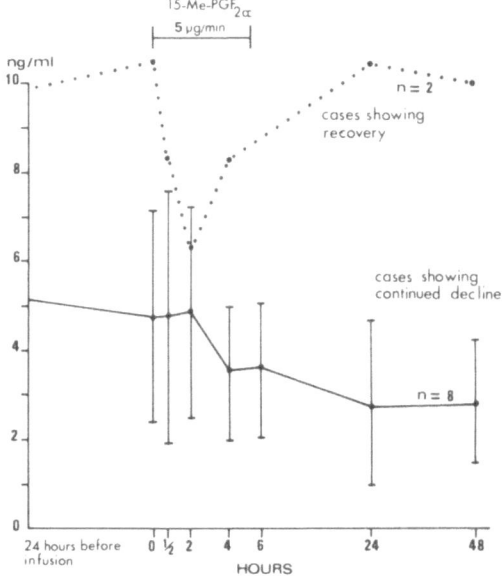

Figure 4.10 Mean plasma progesterone levels ($\pm$ SD) 24 h before, during the PG infusion of 6 h, and 24 and 48 h, after therapy. The upper part of the figure shows the transient luteolytic effect of 4.5 μg/min PGE$_2$ infusion followed by recovery. The lower part of the figure shows the mean for eight subjects who developed sustained luteolysis in response to 5 μg/min of 15-methyl-PGF$_{2\alpha}$ and for the two cases who showed only a transient fall in progesterone level.

induce luteolysis, though dependent in part on PG–receptor binding, may however, require other parameters which may be hormonally mediated. In the subhuman primate, treatment with PGs and estrogens resulted in luteal regression, whereas PGs alone in a similar set-up required much higher doses to induce similar effects (Shaikh, 1972). Moreover, *in vitro* studies demonstrated that $PGF_{2\alpha}$ can induce a luteolytic effect provided that sufficient amounts of norepinephrine were added to the medium (Hamberger *et al.*, 1980).

It may therefore be concluded that certain PGs may after all be luteolytic in the human, particularly in the presence of an optimal humoral milieu, but a more luteal-specific analog is required if a therapeutic agent of practical value is to be identified. A luteolytic agent has for long been a dream of many scientists involved in the area of contraceptive development. Such a compound with minimal side-effects would approach an ideal agent for fertility control and can be administered by one of three approaches:

(1) as a post-coital agent following unprotected intercourse around mid-cycle;

(2) on a monthly basis in the pre-menstrual phase to induce menstrual-like bleeding;

(3) as a post-conceptional agent or menstrual regulator when the menstruation is delayed for few days. In such a case, either suppression of the corpus luteum of pregnancy, or stimulation of uterine activity, or both, would be the mechanism leading to a very early abortion.

Ovulation

The role of prostaglandins in the process of human ovulation is not fully documented, but several observations in primates and subprimates point towards an important role for these compounds in the occurrence of ovulation:

(1) PGs are probably involved in the hypothalamic–pituitary release of gonadotropins, particularly in subprimate animals. The ability of $PGF_{2\alpha}$ and or PGE_1 or PGE_2 to induce a surge in LH has been demonstrated in subprimates and in rhesus monkeys at various stages of the reproductive cycle (Ojeda *et al.*, 1975; McCann *et al.*, 1976). In the rhesus monkey, subcutaneous administration of 5 mg or more of $PGF_{2\alpha}$ during the second half of the menstrual cycle resulted in variable release of LH with several small peaks. Moreover, indomethacin treatment significantly reduced the LH surge induced by estrogens, i.e. blocked the estrogen positive feedback.

The situation in humans is somewhat different; infusions of $PGF_{2\alpha}$ in males and females did not stimulate FSH or LH release except for some transient LH increase when the infusions were administered in the late luteal phase (Hillier *et al.*, 1972; Coudert and Faiman, 1973; Craig, 1975). However, in one study a PGE_2 analog (Sulprostone) was infused in the follicular phase of the human cycle causing a decrease in LH and FSH levels in a significant percentage of subjects (Abdalla *et al.*, 1979). Moreover, a considerable decrease in the level of circulating LH has been reported in women infused with $PGF_{2\alpha}$ at a rate of $50\,\mu g/min$ for 5 h during the luteal phase (Elias *et al.*, 1975).

PG synthesis inhibitors did not alter LH release induced by Gn RH, while a high dose of aspirin in one subject seemed to block the mid-cycle LH peak (Patrona and Serra, 1974; Chaudhuri and Elder, 1976; Greenway and Swerdloff, 1978). The limited penetration of indomethacin into brain tissue may incompletely inhibit PG synthesis and thus one has to be cautious in the interpretation of studies using this PG inhibitor to reveal PG roles in hypothalamic pituitary function. It therefore appears that the role of PGs in the control of human hypothalamic–pituitary function is not an obligatory one, and remains vague and ill-defined. Further investigations are still needed in this area.

(2) Prostaglandin synthesis inhibitors (non-steroidal anti-inflammatory drugs = NSAID) block ovulation in subhuman primates (marmoset and rhesus monkeys) without interfering with luteinization (Wallach *et al.*, 1975a; Maia *et al.*, 1978). $PGF_{2\alpha}$ administration was able to overcome the block produced by indomethacin and restore ovulation (Wallach *et al.*, 1975b). The ovulation inhibition effect is probably mediated through inhibition of ovarian PG synthesis and thus only the mechanical component of the ovulatory process is altered.

In humans, on the other hand, administration of PG synthesis inhibitors did not interfere with ovulation (Chaudhuri and Elder, 1976; Toppozada *et al.*, 1978, 1979). However, whether the given doses of NSAID suppressed ovarian PG synthesis to a degree sufficient to block ovulation was not verified in these studies. The effect of higher doses with measurement of follicular PG levels may provide valuable information in this respect.

(3) The ovarian synthesis of PGs, particularly in maturing follicles, is markedly increased in the pre-ovulatory phase. Levels of $PGF_{2\alpha}$ in venous blood obtained from human ovarian veins draining ovaries with maturing follicles were significantly higher than the blood levels from the inactive sides (Aksel *et al.*, 1977). Also, the concentration of $PGF_{2\alpha}$ in human follicular fluid from pre-ovulatory follicles was several-fold higher than that obtained from less mature follicles (Edwards, 1973; Patwardhan and Lanthier, 1981; Darling *et al.*, 1982). What releases PGs in the human ovary has not been finally resolved, but there is evidence to support a role for LH in this connection (Plunkett *et al.*, 1975). Whether LH-induced PG production is mediated by the second messenger cAMP is a distinct possibility that requires further confirmation. However, one publication failed to demonstrate a correlation between LH and PGs in cultured ovarian tissues of the human (Liedtke and Seifert, 1978).

(4) The ultimate stimulus that precipitates extrusion of the ovum from the ripe Graafian follicle may involve an increase in the intrafollicular pressure or weakening in the follicular wall or both. PGs appear to participate in these mechanisms. Smooth muscle fibers have been demonstrated in the theca externa and cortical stroma of the human ovary (Okamura *et al.*, 1972) and $PGF_{2\alpha}$ has been shown to induce an *in vitro* and *in vivo* increase in the human and monkey intra-ovarian

pressure (Coutinho and Maia, 1971; Virutamasen *et al.*, 1973). PGs produced within the follicle may either increase the pressure of the growing follicle *per se* or reflected in the overall ovarian contractility. Moreover, intra-ovarian administration of $PGF_{2\alpha}$ in humans induced ovarian contractions *in vivo* which were reduced by oral administration of flufenamic acid (Elder and Coutinho, 1977). Several other hormones have been shown to induce a significant increase in intra-ovarian pressure, especially in the periovulatory phase; these included HMG, HCG, LHRH and norepinephrine (Coutinho and Maia, 1972; Virutamasen *et al.*, 1972; Coutinho *et al.*, 1974). The gonadotropin-induced ovarian pressure changes were believed to be key factors in the process of ovulation, particularly in that only one ovary (the one with ripe follicle) usually responded with increased pressure (Coutinho and Maia, 1972). The interaction between PGs and gonadotropins, LHRH or norepinephrine has been documented relative to other reproductive tissues (human myometrium and corpus luteum), where these humoral substances markedly influenced the tissue response to PGs (Hamberger *et al.*, 1980; El-Dakhakhny, 1980; El-Tarahony, 1982).

Weakening of the Graafian follicle wall is a structural change that seems to aid the process of ovum extrusion, as it was demonstrated that animal follicles about to rupture show disintegration and loosening of the collagenous tissue in its wall (Espey, 1967). PGE_2 has been reported to inhibit collagen synthesis in the apex of human ripe follicles; an effect that was not found in non-apical segments of the pre-ovulatory follicle or in less-developed ones (Dennefors *et al.*, 1982). A similar effect of PGs on collagen synthesis within the human non-pregnant cervical connective tissue has also been reported (Norstrom *et al.*, 1981; Wilhelmsson, 1981).

Another possible mechanism causing structural changes that weaken the follicular wall may involve activation of certain collagenolytic enzymes such as protease and collagenase (Beers *et al.*, 1975 and Morales *et al.*, 1978). Rat granulosa cells from follicles about to rupture produce increasing amounts of the enzyme plasminogen activator which converts plasminogen to plasmin that can weaken follicular wall. Inactive granulosa cells do not possess this capacity unless stimulated by FSH, PGE_1 or PGE_2. It appears that prostaglandins represent a solid link between gonadotrophins and tissue response in the various events leading to the mechanical component of the ovulatory process without interfering with luteinization.

References

Abdalla, M. I., Ibrahim, I. I. and Osman, M. I. (1979). Effect of prostaglandin E_2 derivative (Sulprostone) on the pituitary ovarian function in non-pregnant females. In Friebel, K., Schneider, A. and Wurfel, H. (eds.) *International Sulprostone Symposium*. pp. 113–118. Vienna, November, 1978. (Schering AG)

Akerlund, M. (1979). Pathophysiology of dysmenorrhea. *Acta. Obstet. Gynecol.* (Suppl.), **87**, 27–35

Akerlund, M., Andersson, K. E. and Ingmarsson, I. (1976). Effects of terbutaline on myometrial activity, endometrial blood flow and lower abdominal pain in women with primary dysmenorrhea. *Br. J. Obstet. Gynaecol.*, **83**, 673–678

Aksel, S., Shromberg, D. W. and Hammond, C. B. (1977). Prostaglandin $F_{2\alpha}$ production by the human ovary. *Obstet. Gynecol.*, **50**, 347–350.

Beers, W. H., Strickland, S. and Reich, E. (1975). Ovarian plasminogen activator: Relationships to ovulation and hormonal regulation. *Cell*, **6**, 387–397

Bendz, A. (1977). The anatomical basis for a possible counter current exchange mechanism in the human adnex. *Prostaglandins*, **13**, 355–362

Bolognese, R. J. and Corson, S. L. (1973). The effect of vaginally administered prostaglandin $F_{2\alpha}$ on corpus luteum function. *Am. J. Obstet. Gynecol.*, **117**, 240–245

Borda, E. S., Agostini, M. C., Sterin-Speziale, N., Gimeno, M. F. and Gimeno, A. L. (1979). Spontaneous contractile activity of isolated ovarian human vein. A dual influence of prostacyclin (PGI₂). *Prostaglandins*, **18**, 829–835

Bygdeman, M., Fredricsson, B., Svanborg, K. and Samuelsson, B. (1970). The relation between fertility and prostaglandin content of seminal fluid in man. *Fertil. Steril.*, **21**, 622–629

Bygdeman, M., Bremme, K., Gillespie, A. and Lundstrom, V. (1979). Effects of prostaglandins on the uterus. Prostaglandins and uterine contractility. *Acta Obstet. Gynecol. Scand.*, Suppl. **87**, 33–38

Carlson, J. C., Wong, A. P. and Perrin, D. G. (1977). The effects of prostaglandin and mating on release of LH in the female rabbit. *J. Reprod. Fertil.*, **51**, 87–92

Challis, J. R. G., Calder, A. A., Dilley, S., Forster, C. S., Hillier, K., Hunter, D. J. S. Mackenzie, I. Z. and Thorburn, G. D. (1976). Production of prostaglandins E and $F_{2\alpha}$ by corpora lutea, corpora albicantes and stroma from the human ovary. *J. Endocrinol.*, **68**, 401–408

Channing, C. P. (1972). Stimulatory effects of prostaglandins upon luteinization of rhesus monkey granulosa cell cultures. *Prostaglandins*, **2**, 331–349

Chaudhuri, G. and Elder, M. G. (1976). Lack of evidence for inhibition of ovulation by aspirin in women. *Prostaglandins*, **11**, 727–735

Clithero, H. J. and Pickles, V. R. (1961). The separation of the smooth muscle stimulants in menstrual fluid. *J. Physiol. (Lond.)*, **156**, 225–237

Coudert, S. P. and Faiman, C. (1973). Effect of $PGF_{2\alpha}$ on anterior pituitary function in man. *Prostaglandins*, **3**, 89–95

Coudert, S. P., Winter, J. S. D. and Faiman, C. (1974). Transient decline in serum progesterone levels during prostaglandin $F_{2\alpha}$ infusion in the mid-luteal phase of the normal menstrual cycle. *Am. J. Obstet. Gynecol.*, **119**, 755–761

Coutinho, E. M. and Darzé, E. (1976). Spontaneous contractility and the response of the human uterine cervix to prostaglandin $F_{2\alpha}$ and E_2 during the menstrual cycle. *Am. J. Obstet. Gynecol.*, **126**, 224–225

Coutinho, E. M. and Maia, H. (1971). The contractile response of the human uterus, Fallopian tubes, and ovary to prostaglandins *in vivo*. *Fertil. Steril.*, **22**, 539–543

Coutinho, E. M. and Maia, H. S. (1972). Effects of gonadotrophin on motility of human ovary. *Nature New Biol.*, **235**, 94–96

Coutinho, E. M., Maia, H. S. and Schally, A. V. (1974). Changes in intra-ovarian pressure in women following the administration of luteinizing-hormone releasing hormone (LH-RH). *Int. J. Fertil.*, **19**, 89–92

Coyotupa, J., Buster, J., Parlow, A. and Dignam, W. (1973). Normal cyclical patterns of serum gonadotrophins and ovarian steroids despite congenital absence of the uterus. *J. Clin. Endocrinol. Metab.*, **36**, 395–399

Craig, G. M. (1975). The effect of intravenous $PGF_{2\alpha}$ on serum luteinizing hormone, follicle stimulating hormone and plasma cortisol in normal men. *J. Clin. Endocrinol. Metab.*, **41**, 180–182

Csapo, A. I. and Pinto-Dantas, C. R. (1966). The cyclic activity of the non-pregnant uterus, A new method for recording intra-uterine response. *Fertil. Steril.*, **17**, 34–38

Darling, M. R. N., Jogee, M. and Elder, M. G. (1982). Prostaglandin $F_{2\alpha}$ levels in the human ovarian follicle. *Prostaglandins*, **23**, 551–556

Dennefors, B., Tjugum, J., Norstrom, A., Janson, P. O., Nilsson, L., Hamberger, L. and Wilhelmsson, L. (1982). Collagen synthesis inhibition by PGE_2 within the human follicular wall-one possible mechanism underlying ovulation. *Prostaglandins*, **24**, 295–302

Doyle, L. L., Barclay, D. L., Duncan, G. W. and Kirton, K. T. (1971). Human luteal function following hysterectomy as assessed by plasma progestin. *Am. J. Obstet. Gynecol.*, **110**, 92–97

Edwards, R. G. (1973). Studies in human conception. *Am. J. Obstet. Gynecol.*, **117**, 587–601

Einer-Jensen, N. (1973). Decreased endometrial blood flow and plasma progesterone level after instillation of 10 μg $PGF_{2\alpha}$ into the lumen of the uteri of rhesus monkeys. *Prostaglandins*, **4**, 517–533

El-Dakhakhny, M. M. (1980). Response of the non-pregnant human uterus to prostaglandin E_2 and its derivatives under different hormonal conditions. *Ph.D. thesis*. The University of Alexandria, Egypt

Elder, M. G. and Coutinho, E. M. (1977). Human ovarian motility induced by $PGE_{2\alpha}$. Quoted by Darling *et al.* (1982), *Prostaglandins*, **23**, 551

Elias, J. A., Newton, J. R. and Collins, W. P. (1975). Changes in ovarian and pituitary function in non-pregnant women during the infusion of $PGF_{2\alpha}$. *Acta Endocrinol.*, **80**, 676–685

El-Tarahony, A. L. H. (1982). Effect of LHRH and HCG on the uterine response to local PGE_2 in non-pregnant women. *M.S. thesis*, The University of Alexandria, Egypt

Espey, L. L. (1967). Ultrastructure of the rabbit Graafian follicle during the ovulatory process. *Endocrinology*, **81**, 267–276

Filler, W. and Warner, J. (1970). Dysmenorrhoea and its therapy. A uterine contractility study. *Am. J. Obstet. Gynecol.*, **106**, 104–109

Green, K., Samuelsson, B., Carlson, J. and McCracken, J. (1972). Prostaglandin $F_{2\alpha}$ identified as a luteolytic hormone in the sheep. *Fourth International Congress Endocrinol.* Pages 189–203. Excerpta Medica, Amsterdam, International Congress Series 256

Greenway, F. L. and Swerdloff, R. S. (1978). Effect of aspirin on ovulation. *Fertil. Steril.*, **30**, 364–373

Halbert, D. R., Demers, L. M., Fontana, J. and Jones, D. E. D. (1975). Prostaglandin levels in endometrial jet wash specimens in patients with dysmenorrhoea before and after indomethacin therapy. *Prostaglandins*, **10**, 1047–1056

Hamberger, L., Nilsson, L., Dennefors, B., Khan, I. and Sjorgen, A. (1979). Cyclic AMP formation of isolated human corpora lutea in response to HCG-Interference by $PGF_{2\alpha}$. *Prostaglandins*, **17**, 615–621

Hamberger, L., Dennefors, B., Hamberger, B., Janson, P. O., Nilsson, L., Sjorgen, A. and Wiqvist, N. (1980). Is vascular innervation a prerequisite for PG-induced luteolysis in the human corpus luteum? In Samuelsson, B., Ramwell, P. and Pasletti, R. (eds.). *Advances in Prostaglandin and Thromboxane Research*, vol. 8, pp. 1365–1368. (New York: Raven Press)

Henderson, K. M. and McNatty, K. P. (1975). A biochemical hypothesis to explain mechanism of luteal regression. *Prostaglandins*, **9**, 779–797

Henzl, M. R., Ortega, E., Gallegos-Cortes, V., Tomlinson, R. V. and Segre, E. J. (1973). Prostaglandin E_2 and the luteal phase of the menstrual cycle: Effects on blood progesterone, estradiol, cortisol and growth hormone levels. *J. Clin. Encrinol. Metab.*, **36**, 784–787

Hillier, K., Dutton, A., Corker, C. S., Singer, A and Embery, M. P. (1972). Plasma steroid and luteinizing hormone levels during $PGF_{2\alpha}$ administration in luteal phase of menstrual cycle. *Br. Med. J.*, 11 November, 333–336

Itoh, K. and Kunimoto, K. (1982). PG levels in venous plasma at menstrual cycle related to deficient corpus luteum – as a cause of infertility. *Int. Conference on PGs (Abstracts)*, Florence, May 1982, p. 386

Jewelewicz, R., Cantor, B., Dyrenfurth, I., Warren, M. P. and Vande-Wiele, R. L. (1972). Intravenous infusion of $PGF_{2\alpha}$ in the mid-luteal phase in the normal human menstrual cycle. *Prostaglandins*, **1**, 443–451

Jones, G. S. and Wentz, A. C. (1972). The effect of prostaglandin $F_{2\alpha}$ infusion on corpus luteum function. *Am. J. Obstet. Gynecol.*, **114**, 393–404

Karim, S. M. M., Hillier, K., Sommers, K. and Trussell, R. R. (1971). The effects of prostaglandins E_2 and $F_{2\alpha}$ administered by different routes on uterine activity and the cardiovascular system in pregnant and non-pregnant women. *J. Obstet. Gynecol. Br. Commonw.*, **78**, 172–179

Kinoshita, K., Eneroth, P. and Bygdeman, M. (1979). Treatment with a single vaginal suppository containing 15-methyl $PGF_{2\alpha}$ methyl ester at expected time of menstruation. *Prostaglandins*, **17**, 469–481

Kirton, K. T. (1975). Prostaglandins and reproduction in subhuman primates. In Karim, S. M. M. (ed.). *Prostaglandins and Reproduction*, pp. 229–240. (Lancaster: MTP Press)

Korda, A. R., Shutt, D. A., Smith, I. D., Shearman, R. P. and Lyneham, R. C. (1975). Assessment of possible luteolytic effect of intra-ovarian injection of Prostaglandin $F_{2\alpha}$ in the human. *Prostaglandins*, **9**, 443–449

Leader, A., Bygdeman, M., Eneroth, P., Martin, J. N. Jr. and Wiqvist, N. (1976). The effect of infusion with two analogues of prostaglandins $F_{2\alpha}$ on corpus luteum function. In Samuelsson, B. and Paoletti, R. (eds.). *Advances in Prostaglandins and Thromboxane Research.* Vol. 2, pp. 679–684 (New York: Raven Press)

Lehmann, F., Peters, F., Breckwoldt, M. and Bettendorf, G. (1972). Plasma progesterone levels during infusion of $PGF_{2\alpha}$ in the human. *Prostaglandins*, **1**, 269–277

Lemaire, W. J. and Shapiro, W. G. (1972). Prostaglandin $F_{2\alpha}$. Its effect on the corpus luteum of the menstrual cycle. *Prostaglandins*, **1**, 259–267

Liedtke, M. P. and Seifert, B. (1978). Biosynthesis of prostaglandins in human ovarian tissues. *Prostaglandins*, **16**, 825–833

Lundstrom, V. (1977). The myometrial response to intra-uterine administration of $PGF_{2\alpha}$ and PGE_2 in dysmenorrheic women. *Acta Obstet. Gynecol. Scand.*, **56**, 167–172

Lundstrom, V. and Green, K. (1978). Endogenous levels of prostaglandin $F_{2\alpha}$ and its main metabolites in plasma and endometrium of normal and dysmenorrhoic women. *Am. J. Obstet. Gynecol.*, **130**, 640–646

Lundstrom, V., Green, K. and Wiqvist, N. (1976). Prostaglandins, indomethacin and dysmenorrhea. *Prostaglandins*, **11**, 893–904

Lundstrom, V., Green, K. and Svanborg, K. (1979). Endogenous prostaglandins in dysmenorrhoea and the effect of prostaglandin synthetase inhibitor on uterine contractility. *Acta Obstet. Gynecol. Scand.*, Suppl. **87**, 51–56

Lyneham, R. C., Korda, A. R., Shutt, D. A., Smith, I. D. and Shearman, R. P. (1975). The effect of intrauterine prostaglandin $F_{2\alpha}$ on corpus luteum function in the human. *Prostaglandins*, **9**, 431–442

Maathuis, J. B. and Kelly, R. W. (1978). Prostaglandin $F_{2\alpha}$ and E_2 in the endometrium throughout the menstrual cycle, after the administration of clomiphene or an estrogen-progestogen pill and in early pregnancy. *J. Endocrinol.*, **77**, 361–371

Maia, H., Barbosa, I. and Coutinho, E. M. (1978). Inhibition of ovulation in marmoset monkeys by indomethacin. *Fertil. Steril.*, **29**, 565–570

Mann, E. C., Thomas, C. L. and Carmichael, D. E. (1962). Myometrial and isthmic mechanisms in primary dysmenorrhea. *Obstet. Gynecol.*, **13**, 408–414

Marsh, J. M. and Lemaire, W. J. (1974). Cyclic AMP accumulation and steroidogenesis in human corpus luteum. Effect on gonadotrophins and prostaglandins. *J. Clin. Endocrinol. Metab.*, **38**, 99–106

Martin, J. N. Jr., Bygdeman, M. and Eneroth, P. (1978). The influence of locally administered prostaglandin E_2 and $F_{2\alpha}$ on uterine motility in the intact non-pregnant human uterus. *Acta Obstet. Gynecol. Scand.*, **57**, 141–147

McCann, S. M., Ojeda, S. R., Harms, P. G., Wheaton, J. E. Sundberg, D. J. T. and Fawcett, C. P. (1976). In Naftolin, F., Ryan, K. J. and Davies, J., (eds). *Subcellular Mechanisms in Reproductive Neuroendocrinology.* pp. 407–422. (Amsterdam: Elsevier)

McCracken, J. (1971). Prostaglandins and corpus luteum regression. *Ann. N.Y. Acad. Sci.*, **180**, 456–472

Morales, T. I., Woessner, J. F., Howell, D. S., Marsh, J. M. and LeMaire, W. J. (1978). A microassay for the direct demonstration of collagenolytic activity in graafian follicles of the rat. *Biochim. Biophys. Acta*, **524**, 428–434

Norstrom, A., Wilhelmsson, L. and Hamberger, L. (1981). The regulatory influence of prostaglandins on protein synthesis on the human non-pregnant cervix. *Prostaglandins*, **22**, 117–124

Ojeda, S. R., Wheaton, J. E. and McCann, S. M. (1975). Prostaglandin E_2 induced release of luteinizing hormone releasing factor (LRF). *Neuroendocrinology*, **17**, 283–287

Okamura, H., Aso., T., Yoshida, Y. and Nishimure, T. (1974). Effect of prostaglandin $F_{2\alpha}$ on human corpora lutea. *Obstet. Gynecol. NY*, **44**, 127–134

Okamura, H., Virutamasen, P., Wright, K. H. and Wallach, E. E. (1972). Ovarian smooth muscle in the human being, rabbit and cat. Histochemical and electron microscopic study. *Am. J. Obstet. Gynecol.*, **112**, 183–191

Patrona, C. and Serra, G. B. (1974). Do pituitary prostaglandins play an essential role in the action of LHRH in man. *Prostaglandins*, **6**, 345–346

Patwardhan, V. V. and Lanthier, A. (1974). Effect of prostaglandins on the *in vitro* steroidogenesis in human ovarian tissues. *Prostaglandins*, **6**, 385–388

Patwardhan, V. V. and Lanthier, A. (1980). Concentrations of prostaglandins PGE and PGF, estrone, estradiol and progesterone in human corpora lutea. *Prostaglandins*, **20**, 963–969

Patwardhan, V. V. and Lanthier, A. (1981). Prostaglandins PGE and PGF in human ovarian follicles: Endogenous contents and in vitro formation by theca and granulosa cells. *Acta Endocrinol. (Copenh).*, **97**, 543–550

Pickles, V. R. (1959). Myometrial responses to the menstrual plain muscle stimulant. *J. Endocrinol.*, **19**, 150–157

Pickles, V. R., Hall, W. J., Best, F. A. and Smith, G. N. (1965). Prostaglandins in endometrium and menstrual fluid from normal and dysmenorrhoeic subjects. *J. Obstet. Gynaecol. Br. Commonw.*, **72**, 185–192

Plunkett, E. R., Moon, Y. S., Zamecnik, J. and Armstrong, D. T. (1975). Preliminary evidence of a role for prostaglandin F in human follicular function. *Am. J. Obstet. Gynecol.*, **123**, 391–397

Powell, W. S., Hammarstrom, S. and Samuelsson, B. (1974). Prostaglandin $F_{2\alpha}$ receptor in human corpora lutea. *Lancet*, **1**, 1120

Poyser, N. L. (1981). Prostaglandins in reproduction. In Bakhle, Y. S. (ed.), *Research Studies Press.* p. 108 (Chichester: John Wiley)

Pulkkinen, M. O. (1979). Suppression of uterine activity by prostaglandin synthetase inhibitors. *Acta Obstet. Gynecol. Scand.*, **87**, 39–43

Pulkkinen, M. O., Henzl, M. R. and Csapo, M. I. (1978). The effect of Naproxen-sodium on the prostaglandin concentrations of the menstrual blood and uterine 'jet-washings' in dysmenorrheic women. *Prostaglandins*, **15**, 543–550

Rahman, H. A., El-Sokkary, H. A., El-Abd, M. M., Shaala, S. A., Gaweesh, S. S. and Toppozada, M. K. (1982). Transient luteolytic effect of prostaglandins E_2 in humans. *Asia-Oceania J. Obstet. Gynaecol.*, **8**, 413–417

Rosenwaks, Z. and Jones, G. (1980). Menstrual pain: its origin and pathogenesis. *J. Reprod. Med.* **25** (Suppl. 4), 207–211

Roth-Brandel, V., Bygdeman, M. and Wiqvist, N. (1970). Effect of intravenous administration of prostaglandin E_1 and $F_{2\alpha}$ on the contractility of the non-pregnant human uterus in vivo. *Acta Obstet. Gynecol. Scand.*, **49**, (Suppl. 5), 19–41

Russell, W. (1975). Luteolysis induced in pigtail monkeys (*Macaca nemestrina*) with prostaglandin $F_{2\alpha}$ ICI 80996 and ICI 81008. *Prostaglandins*, **10**, 163–183

Saleh, A. (1982). Effect of thromboxane B_2 on the non-pregnant human uterus. *M.S. thesis.* The University of Alexandria, Egypt

Salem, A. I. S. (1982). Effect of prostaglandins and their synthesis inhibitors on uterine activity in primary dysmenorrhoea. *M.D. thesis*, The University of Alexandria, Egypt

Schick, B. (1920). Das menstruationsgift. *Wien Klin. Wochenschr.*, **19**, 1. Quoted by Pickles, V. R. (1978). Prostaglandins and dysmenorrhoea, *Acta Obstet. Gynecol.*, Suppl. **87**, 7–12

Shaala, S., Gaafar, A. and Toppozada, M. (1974). Response of the menopausal uterus to prostaglandins. In Toppozada, M. (ed.) *Prostaglandins in Human Reproduction*, pp. 95–102. (Alexandria: Alexandria University Press)

Shaala, S., Khowessah, M., El-Damarawy, H., El-Sahwi, S. and Toppozada, M. (1977). Reduced uterine response to $PGF_{2\alpha}$ under oral contraceptives. *Prostaglandins*, **14**, 523–533

Shaala, S., El-Damarawy, H., Gaafar, T. E. and Toppozada, M. (1983). Effect of the main metabolite of prostacyclin on the contractility of the non-pregnant uterus, prostaglandins, *Leukotriens and Medicine* (In press)

Shaikh, A. A. (1972). Regulation of menstrual cycle and termination of pregnancy in the monkey by estradiol and $PGF_{2\alpha}$. *Prostaglandins*, **2**, 227–233

Shutt, D. A., Clarke, A. H., Fraser, I. S., Goh, P., McMahon, G. R., Saunders, D. M. and Shearman, R. P. (1976). Changes in concentration of prostaglandin F and steroids in human corpora lutea in relation to growth of the corpus luteum and luteolysis. *J. Endocrinol.*, **71**, 453–456

Sun, F. F., Chapman, J. P. and McGuire, J. C. (1977). Metabolism of prostaglandin endoperoxide in animal tissues. *Prostaglandins*, **14**, 1055–1074

Svanborg, K., Bendvold, E., Bygdeman, M. and Eneroth, P. (1982). The relation between PGs in human seminal fluid and fertility. *Int. Conference on PGs (Abst.)* Florence, May 1982, p. 711

Swanston, I. A., McNatty, K. P. and Baird, D. T. (1977). Concentration of Prostaglandin $F_{2\alpha}$ and steroids in the human corpus luteum. *J. Endocrinol.*, **73**, 115–122

Swahn, M. L. and Lundstrom, V. (1983). The effect of intravenous and intrauterine administration of prostacyclin on the non-pregnant uterine contractility in vivo. *Acta Obstet Gynecol. Scand.*, Suppl. **113**, 47–50

Tom, W. K. C., Thorneycroft, J. H., Nakamura, R. M. and Mishell, D. R. Jr (1972). Intravaginal $PGF_{2\alpha}$ as a luteolytic agent. Advanced abstracts, p. 110. International Conference on Prostaglandins, Vienna, September 1972. (Oxford: Pergamon Press Vieweg)

Toppozada, M. (1975). Letter to the editor. *Prostaglandins*, **10**, 725

Toppozada, M. and Hafez, E. S. E. (1980). The role of prostaglandins in the mechanism of action and side-effects of IUD. In E. S. E. Hafez and Van Os, W. A. A. (eds). *Medicated Intrauterine Devices*, pp. 84–98. (Amsterdam: Martinus Nijhoff)

Toppozada, M., Gaafar, A. and Shaala, S. (1974a). *In vivo* inhibition of the human non-pregnant uterus by prostaglandin E_2. *Prostaglandins*, **8**, 401–410

Toppozada, M., Beguin, F., Bygdeman, M. and Wiqvist, N. (1972). Response of the mid-pregnant human uterus to systemic administration of 15 (s) methyl $PGF_{2\alpha}$. *Prostaglandins*, **2**, 239–249

Toppozada, M., Rizk, M. A. and El-Agouz, W. (1974b). Corpus luteum demise by prostaglandin $F_{2\alpha}$. In Toppozada, M. (ed.) *Prostaglandins in Human Reproduction*. pp. 85–93. (Alexandria: Alexandria University Press)

Toppozada, M., Gaafar, A., Shaala, S. and Osman, M. (1975). The relaxant property of local prostaglandin E_2 on the non-pregnant uterus – A cyclic triphasic response. *Prostaglandins*, **9**, 475–486

Toppozada, M., Khowessah, M., Shaala, S., Said, S. and Osman, M. (1976). Uterine response to prostaglandin E_2 under oral contraceptives. *Contraception*, **13**, 749–761

Toppozada, M., Khowessah, M., Shaala, S., Osman, M. and Rahman, H. A. (1977). Aberrant uterine response to prostaglandin E_2 as a possible etiologic factor in functional infertility. *Fertil. Steril.*, **28**, 434–439

Toppozada, M., Khalil, T. H. and El-Sokkary, H. (1978). The role of prostaglandins in the control of human pituitary ovarian function. *Proc. 6th. Asia and Oceania Congress of Endocrinology*, pp. 143–151. 22–27 January Singapore

Toppozada, M., El-Abd, M., El-Sokkary, H., El-Rahman, H. A., Khalil, T. H. and Galal, R. (1979). Effect of a prostaglandin inhibitor on human ovulation. *Sing. J. Obstet. Gynaecol.*, **10**, 42–46

Toppozada, M., Rizk, M., Thabet, M. H. and Shaala, S. (1980). Uterine response to PGE_2 with IUDs: a possible mechanism of action and side-effects. *Contracept. Deliv. Syst.*, **1**, 349–361

Toppozada, M., El-Sokkary, H., El-Abd, M., El-Fazary, A. and El-Rahman, H. (1981). Induction of human luteolysis by high dose infusions of 15-methyl $PGF_{2\alpha}$. *Prostaglandins Med.*, **6**, 203–211

Toppozada, M., Shaala, S., Saleh, A. and Damarawy, H. (1983). Effect of thromboxane B_2 on the contractility of the non-pregnant human uterus. *Prostaglandins, Leukotriens Med.* (In press)

Virutamasen, P., Wright, K. H. and Wallach, E. E. (1972). Effects of catecholamines on ovarian contractility in the rabbit. *Obstet. Gynecol.*, **39**, 225–236

Virutamasen, P., Wright, K. H. and Wallach, E. E. (1973). Monkey ovarian contractility – its relationship to ovulation. *Fertil. Steril.*, **24**, 763–771

Wallach, E. E., de la Cruz, A., Hunt, J., Wright, K. and Stevens, V. C. (1975a). The effect of indomethacin on HMG–HCG induced ovulation in the rhesus monkey. *Prostaglandins*, **9**, 645–658

Wallach, E. E., Bronson, R., Hamada, Y., Wright, K. and Stevens, V. C. (1975b). Effectiveness of $PGF_{2\alpha}$ in restoration of HMG–HCG induced ovulation in indomethacin treated rhesus monkeys. *Prostaglandins*, **10**, 129–138

Wentz, A. C. and Jones, G. S. (1972). Effect of infused $PGF_{2\alpha}$ on human corpus luteum function and menses. *Brook Lodge Symposium on Prostaglandins*. (Abst.) June 1972, p. 47

Wentz, A. C. and Jones, G. S. (1973). Transient luteolytic effect of $PGF_{2\alpha}$ in humans. *Obstet. Gynecol.*, **42**, 172–181

Wilhelmsson, L., Lindblom, B. and Wiqvist, N. (1979). The human uterotubal junction. Contractile patterns of different smooth muscle layers and influence of PGE_2, $PGF_{2\alpha}$ and PGI_2 in vitro. *Fertil. Steril*, **32**, 303–307

Wilhelmsson, L. (1981). Biological actions of prostaglandins on different tissues within the non-pregnant human uterus. *M.D. thesis.* Department of Obstetrics and Gynecology, University of Göteborg, Sweden, pp. 1–44

Wilhelmsson, L., Wikland, M. and Wiqvist, N. (1981). PGH_2, $Tx\ A_2$ and PGI_2 have potent and differentiated actions on human uterine contractility. *Prostaglandins*, **21**, 277–286

Wiqvist, N. and Wilhelmsson, L. (1979). Some clinical and theoretical aspects on prostaglandins in Obstetrics and Gynecology. *Gynecol. Obstet. Invest.*, **10**, 1–8

Wiqvist, N., Bygdeman, M. and Kirton, K. T. (1971). Non-steroidal antifertility agents in the female. In Diczfalusy, E. and Borell, U. (eds.). *Nobel Symposium 15: Control of Human Fertility.* pp. 137–155. (Stockholm: Almqvist & Wiksell)

5
Prostaglandin-induced changes in the pregnant human cervix

W. RATH, P. THEOBALD, H. KÜHNLE, and W. KUHN

CLINICAL ASPECTS OF LOCAL PG ADMINISTRATION

The ability of prostaglandins (PGs) to induce labor in the human led in the late 1960s to highly efficient methods for induction of abortion in the first and second trimesters (Bydgeman et al., 1968; Karim et al., 1968). Since then, PGs have been used by various routes for induction of labor (review by Karim et al., 1979). In some cases the application of PGs resulted in favorable cervical scores without onset of labor (Haspels and Neth, 1973; Toppozada et al., 1973), which would suggest that cervical ripening may occur independent of prominent uterine contractions (Stys et al., 1978; Ulmsten, 1979).

The extra-amniotic administration of PG, either by a continuous infusion or by a single or repeated injection of PG in a viscous gel, has shown promising results both for ripening of the cervix and for induction of labor (review by MacKenzie, 1981). Intracervical instillation of PG gel aims at administering PG as near as possible to the target organ, and has been successfully employed either for ripening the cervix prior to surgical evacuation of the uterus in first trimester abortions (Kühnle et al., 1977) or for treatment of the unfavorable cervix before induction of labor at term (Steiner et al., 1979; Ulmsten, 1979).

Radiological methods proved that the gel was well located within the cervical canal (Ulmsten and Wingerup, 1980) and its high viscosity prevents leakage from the cervical canal (Lippert, 1979). Previous double blind studies have confirmed that the PG, and not the gel-vehicle *per se* or its application, was responsible for ripening the cervix (Wingerup et al., 1979; Ulmsten et al., 1979). Since 1975 the intracervical application of self-developed PG gel has proved to be a safe and practicable method to soften and dilate the cervix in more than 2500 first trimester abortions in our clinic (Rath et al., 1982). The beneficial softening effect of locally applied PG cannot be explained without referral to fundamental mechanical, histological and biochemical changes in the uterine cervix.

PHYSICAL INVESTIGATIONS

Changes in the physical properties of the pregnant cervix after PG treatment

Prostaglandins cause increased distensibility of cervical tissue both *in vitro* and *in vivo* in man and other mammals (Liggins, 1978). The administration of PG directly into the cervical lumen of late-pregnant ewes produced softening, shortening and dilatation of the cervix (Liggins, 1978; Fitzpatrick, 1977). PGE has been shown to have a direct local action on the pregnant rat cervix, causing increased extensibility (Hollingsworth, 1981). The stretch modulus of human cervical tissue *in vitro* is increased approximately 50 % during incubation with $PGF_{2\alpha}$ and to a lesser extent with PGE_2 (Conrad and Ueland, 1976). Results obtained from these experimental studies are in accordance with clinical observations suggesting a reduction of the tissue firmness and a dilatation of the cervix after local administration of PG (review by MacKenzie, 1981).

Evaluation of the amount or degree of cervical softening and dilatation has been hampered by the lack of any objective method of measurements of these parameters, and usually has been based only on the subjective estimate of the operators (Dingfelder *et al.*, 1975). The extreme variability of force applied by different operators in dilating the cervix has been pointed out (Hulka *et al.*, 1974). Our studies have aimed at obtaining objective criteria for the dilating effect of locally applied PG.

Objective demonstration of cervical softening with a PG gel

Abortion was induced in 100 patients during the 7th to 13th week of gestation by intracervical application of $PGF_{2\alpha}$ gel. The gel consisted of 3ml 5 % Tylose containing 3 mg $PGF_{2\alpha}$. A cervical tonometer was constructed which permits precise objective measurements of the resistance force encountered during cervical dilatation (Fig. 5.1). The tonometer consists of modified Hegar dilators and a spring balance which determines the highest resistance by means of a scale. The latter is divided into 12 units, each of which corresponds to 160 pond. One person was solely responsible for the readings. The resistance force of the cervical canal (at the isthmus) was measured on four separate occasions: before PG gel application, at operation 6–8 h after PG treatment, and on the 4th day and 5–6 weeks after abortion. Evacuation of the uterus was performed under general anesthesia by instrumental curettage.

At operation 6–8 h after intracervical PG administration the cervix proved to be freely passable (i.e. below 160 pond) for at least Hegar 8 in 99 % of patients. Lower resistance was encountered in multigravidae than in primigravidae; 57 % of primigravidae and 74 % of multigravidae were dilatable to Hegar 10 (Fig. 5.2). The extent of dilatation increased proportionally with the duration of pregnancy. The cervix was dilated up to Hegar 10 in 72 % of the patients between the 10th and 12th week, whereas this was observed in only 45.5 % between the 7th and 9th week of gestation.

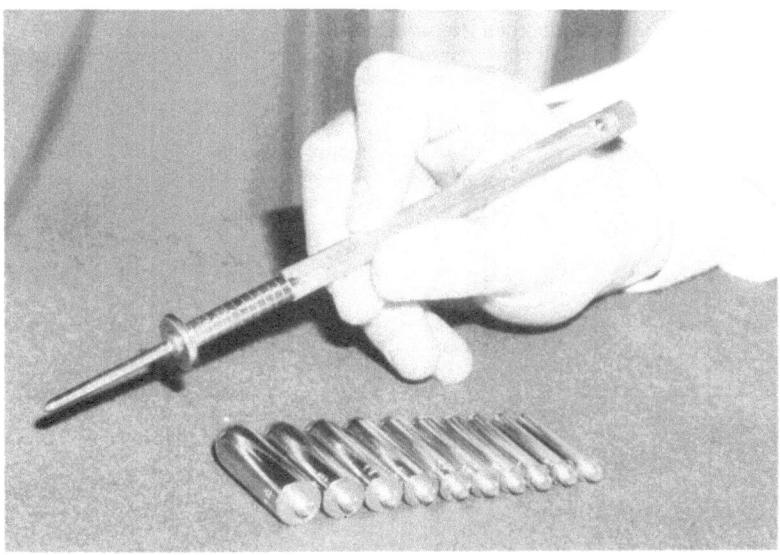

Figure 5.1 The complete tonometer ready for use

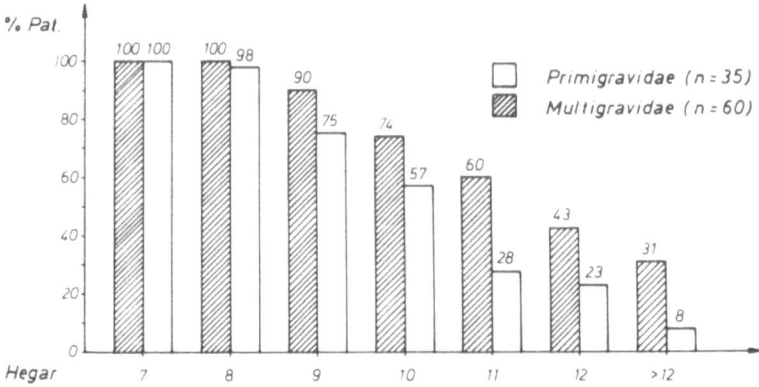

Figure 5.2 Free passability of the cervix after $PGF_{2\alpha}$ gel application in primi- and multigravidae related to different Hegar dilators

The resistance of the cervical canal was the same prior to gel application and 5–6 weeks after abortion in 92 % of the patients. This was measured with Hegar dilators No. 4 (Table 5.1). There were no spontaneous or operation-induced cervical lesions; however, the softened cervix seemed susceptible to tenaculum laceration.

Similar force-measuring dilators have been used to determine the resistance force encountered during cervical dilatation (Liu *et al.*, 1975; Calder, 1981). A

Table 5.1 Mean values of cervical resistance before PGE application, 6–8 h after, and on the 4th day and 4–6 weeks after abortion (Hegar dilators No. 4)

Patients	n	Before PG application	6–8 h after PG application	4 days after PG application	5–6 weeks after PG application (n = 96*)
Nulliparae	60	488 p	< 160 p	264 p	464 p (n = 58)
Nulliparae with previous interruption	3	368 p	< 160 p	160 p	368 p (n = 3)
Multiparae	35	352 p	< 160 p	264 p	416 p (n = 33)
Multiparae with previous interruption	2	320 p	< 160 p	240 p	240 p (n = 2)
	100	382 p	< 160 p	232 p	372 p (n = 96)

p = Pond.
* = Four cases lost to follow-up.

so-called 'Electronic Force Monitor' was described by Hulka *et al.* (1974) and was used by Dingfelder *et al.* (1975) to measure objectively the dilating effect of $PGF_{2\alpha}$ in pregnant women. Patients receiving $PGF_{2\alpha}$ vaginal suppositories exhibited greatly reduced cervical resistance.

In a comparison between $PGF_{2\alpha}$ and PGE_2 suppositories PGE_2 has been shown to be less effective in reducing the force needed for dilatation (Dingfelder *et al.*, 1975). On the other hand, results obtained from experimental studies using the modified method of Harkness and Harkness (1959) demonstrated a higher dilating efficiency of PGE_2 (Lippert *et al.*, 1982).

Before induction of labor, PGE_2 seems to be a more potent agent than $PGF_{2\alpha}$ for ripening the human uterine cervix (MacKenzie and Embrey, 1979).

Although the efficacy of locally applied prostaglandins may depend to an extent on their ability to stimulate uterine activity the results of clinical studies suggest that PGs exert direct effects on the cervical connective tissue.

HISTOLOGICAL CHANGES IN THE CONNECTIVE TISSUE OF THE CERVIX DURING PREGNANCY AND LABOR

Dilatation of the cervix is an active, dynamic process involving fundamental changes within the tissue structure of the cervix (Veis, 1980). The ultrastructure of the non-pregnant cervix is dominated by densely wavy and sometimes intertwined collagen fibers (Danforth *et al.*, 1960). The collagen fibers have a periodicity of 640 Å, suggesting a constant amino acid sequence and an intact polypeptide chain (Buckingham *et al.*, 1962). In the second half of pregnancy the collagen fibers change from compact bundles to a loosely arranged network as parturition approaches.

At the end of labor the collagen fibers are reduced in size and become highly branched (Danforth *et al.*, 1960). There seems to be a dissociation of the collagen bundles into their fibrillar components, which appears to be the fundamental change being responsible for the increasing effacement and dilatability of the cervix (Liggins, 1978).

The increasing dilatability of the cervix and its complete dilatation in labor do not necessarily involve any alteration of the natural state of collagen, as evidenced by the persistence of the 640 Å banding (Buckingham *et al.*, 1962). Electron microscopic studies demonstrated a marked reduction of collagen fibers in the intrapartum cervix (Junquira *et al.*, 1980) and an increase of the interfibrillar substance in humans (Berwind, 1954) as well as in rats (Bryant *et al.*, 1968). Like the physiological maturation around the time of delivery, cervical maturation may be induced by local administration of PG.

The study which follows was aimed at elucidating in which way locally applied PGs act on the collagenous connective tissue of the uterine cervix.

Histological changes in the connective tissue of the pregnant PG-treated cervix, in comparison with the non-pregnant cervix and cervix of early pregnancy

For examination by light microscopy biopsies were taken to a depth of 5–10 mm from the posterior lip of:

(a)   14 non-pregnant patients of childbearing age;
(b)   7 women having a pregnancy termination at 9–14 weeks gestation;
(c)   6 women having a termination of pregnancy (9–13 weeks) who had had an intracervical PG gel ($PGF_{2\alpha}$) instillation 8 h previously.

Serial sections were prepared and stained with trichrome according to Masson to demonstrate the collagen fibers. Collagen fibers show up after trichrome staining as a bright green fibrous network.

The non-pregnant cervix

This typically shows densely packed and finely wavy collagen fibers (Fig. 5.3A). The collagen appears as highly woven bundles of interlacing bright green fibers as described by Danforth *et al.* (1960, 1974).

In the pregnant cervix

Here the collagen fibers are less densely packed and the waves are broader and deeper. The fibers are sometimes twisted and the density of their packing varied (Fig. 5.3B).

In the pregnant PG-treated cervix

Here these changes become even more marked. The collagen fibers are looser, dissociated and much more separated from one another so that there are clear spaces filled with fluid between the bundles. The prominent histological feature is that some bunched fibers split into fibrils (Fig. 5.3C) as observed in specimens obtained at term (Fig. 5.3D).

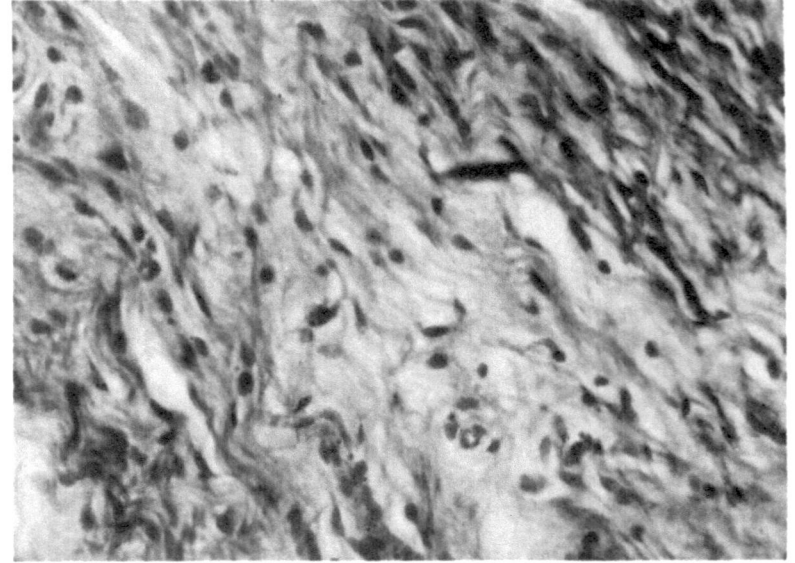

A

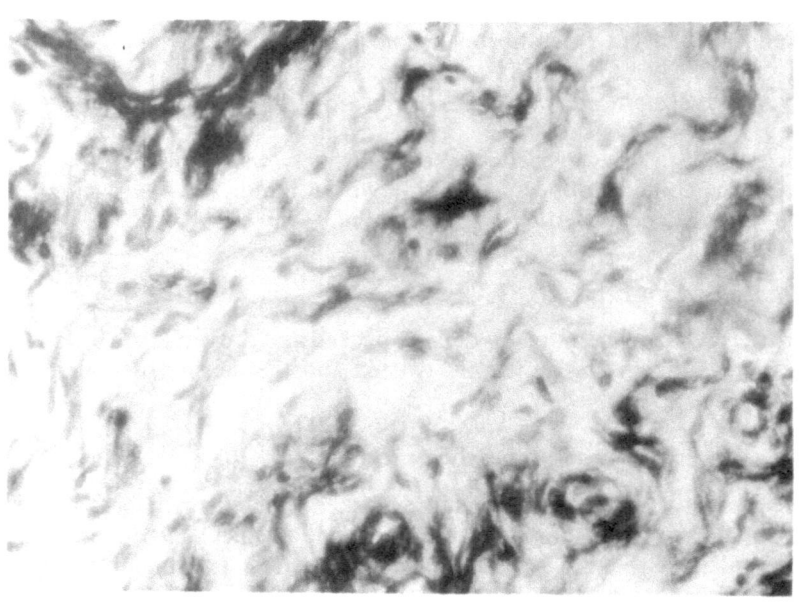

B

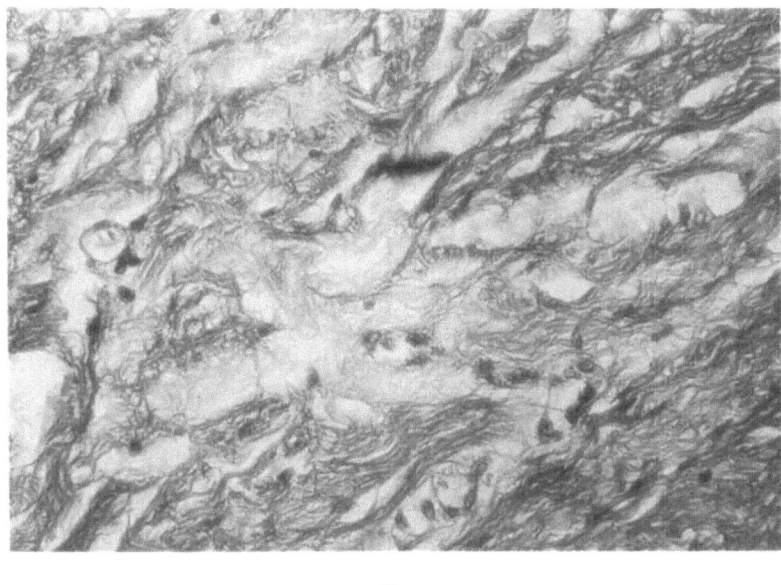

C

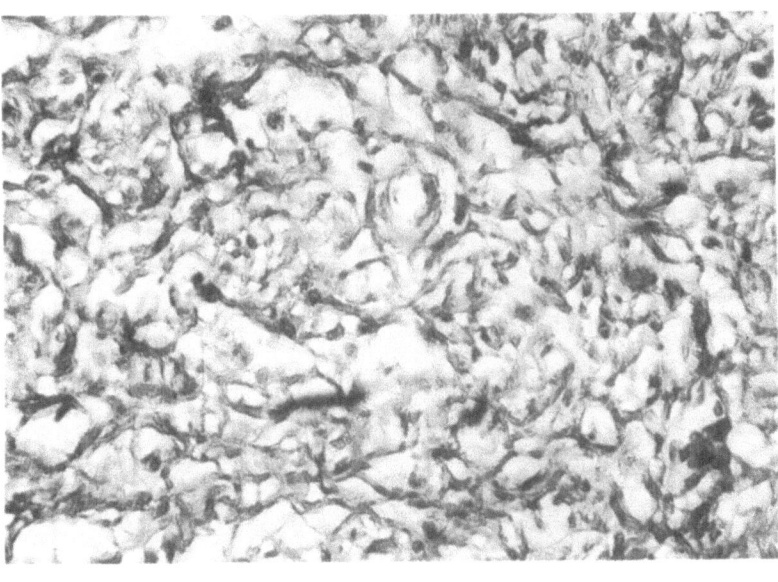

D

Figure 5.3 Serial sections of cervical connective tissue (A–D). A = Collagenous connective tissue of the non-pregnant cervix, without PG (× 162); B = collagenous connective tissue of the pregnant cervix, 12 weeks gestation, without PG (× 216); C = collagenous connective tissue of the pregnant PG-treated cervix (× 216); D = collagenous connective tissue of the pregnant cervix at term (× 216)

Electron microscopic examinations

For electron microscopy, biopsies were taken from five pregnant women at 9–12 weeks gestation (three of whom had been treated with PG gel) and from one non-pregnant patient. These samples were stored in 2% glutaraldehyde solution (0.15M phosphate buffer, pH 7.2).

After PG treatment the fibrils showed a periodicity of 640 Å which is typical for collagen (Fig. 5.4). In some cases electron microscopy showed evidence for the presence of cleavage products.

In conclusion, PG-induced ripening of the cervix is manifested in ultra-structural changes throughout the collagenous connective tissue which are similar to those observed in the ripened cervix at the time of delivery. The presence of cleavage products seems to be associated with the splitting and break-up of the collagen fibrils. These morphological phenomena support the theory of PG-induced collagen breakdown.

Recently the stimulating effect of PG on ripening of the uterine cervix has been investigated by electron microscopy on non-pregnant castrated and pregnant rats (Saito *et al.*, 1981). After intravenous administration of PGE_2 in pregnant rats, collagenous microfibrils increased considerably and collagen fiber bundles showed a considerable tendency to loosen and dissociate (Takahashi *et al.*, 1978; Saito *et al.*, 1981). It was verified from these findings

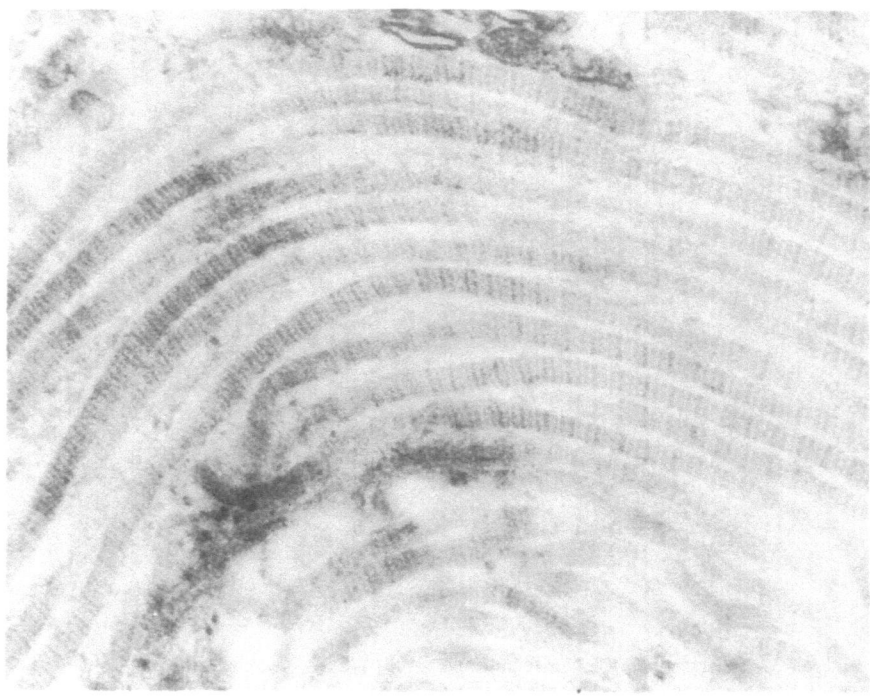

Figure 5.4 Scanning electron micrograph of the collagen fibrils, 10 weeks gestation, 8 h after PG treatment (× 75,000)

that the maturation mechanism of PGE_2 on the pregnant cervix is significantly associated with the 'collagen-dissociation' phenomenon (Takahashi *et al.*, 1978). Electron microscopic studies of human cervical tissue following intracervical PGE_2 gel application have shown dispersal and disintegration of the collagen fibers and a pronounced increase in the amount of ground substance (Uldbjerg *et al.*, 1981). These morphological findings agree well with our results using $PGF_{2\alpha}$ gel. In this context interest has been focused on the fibroblast which is the main source of most connective tissue components and may therefore control the biophysical properties of the connective tissue (Norström *et al.*, 1981).

Probably the mechanism of cervical ripening depends on an altered activity of the fibroblast. However, the stimulus to fibroblasts that promotes these changes is still unknown (Liggins, 1978).

Cervical fibroblasts from subjects treated with PG appear ultrastructurally 'activated' with dispersed nuclear chromatin and proliferation of various cell organelles (Saito *et al.*, 1981; Norström, 1982). These pharmacologically induced morphological effects, similar to those appearing in fibroblasts at parturition (Parry *et al.*, 1981), occur in parallel with a quantitatively and qualitatively altered composition of collagen and ground substance (Norström, 1982). It has been postulated that PGs may modulate the potential of fibroblasts to decrease or increase their ability to synthesize collagen (Norström *et al.*, 1981).

Biochemical changes in the connective tissue of the cervix during pregnancy and labor

Biochemical studies have complemented the histological observations, showing changes in both the collagenous framework and ground substance components of the tissue as the cervix softens (Parry *et al.*, 1981).

In all species studied cervical collagen, extrapolated from the hydroxyproline percentages of the dry weight, decline during pregnancy, indicating either an absolute loss of collagen or a 'dilution' by other connective-tissue components (review by Ellwood, 1981 and Veis, 1980).

The concentration of this amino acid reflects quite accurately the collagen concentration, since in humans it is by and large present only in the collagen molecule or its breakdown products (Maillot *et al.*, 1981). Whereas collagen constitutes 82% of the protein in the non-pregnant cervix, it makes up only 52% at term (Danforth *et al.*, 1974). In addition, there is a marked increase in collagen solubility, suggesting that collagen breakdown occurs parallel to the dilatation of the cervix (review by Maillot *et al.*, 1981). The human cervix at delivery contains few intact collagen chains and hydroxyproline appears to be contained in peptide fragments of collagen molecules arising from active collagenolysis (Kleissl *et al.*, 1978). *In vitro* studies of cervix explants showed evidence for the activity of collagenolytic enzymes involved in the breakdown of the collagen framework (Hillier and Wallis, 1981). However, preliminary attempts to find increased collagenase activity in the maximally dilated human cervix have yielded negative results (Kleissl *et al.*, 1978). Effacement and dilatation of the cervix may be results of proteolytic depolymerization of the fibrils system, and it appears to take place without increase in a specific collagenolytic activity (Veis, 1980). Consequently attention has been focused not on the collagenase, but on the determination of neutral protease and protease inhibitor systems (review by Mori et al., 1981).

Apart from changes in cervical collagen, there are also changes in the main constituents of the ground substance (proteoglycans), which are polysaccharide–protein complexes in which the glycosaminoglycans represent the polysaccharide part of the molecule (Maillot et al., 1979, 1981).

The interrelationship between collagen and glycosaminoglycans has a significant influence on the physical properties of the tissue (Golichowski, 1980). Cervical softening is associated with an increase in the amount of proteoglycans (Danforth et al., 1974; Maillot et al., 1979). Studies of the distribution pattern of glycosaminoglycans have revealed a fall in dermatan sulfate and an increase in hyaluronic acid concentration. The fall in dermatan sulfate is closely related to the fall in cervical collagen concentration throughout gestation (review by Cabrol et al., 1981). These changes would be expected to result in less tightly bound collagen fibrils as observed in morphological investigations (Hillier and Wallis, 1981).

Despite the gross changes in cervical tissue in response to PG, biochemical studies have failed to reveal changes in the content of collagen or in the glycosaminoglycans (Liggins, 1978). A review of our recent published studies relating to the effect of locally applied PG on the hydroxyproline content of the pregnant cervix is presented in the following section.

Biochemical changes in the connective tissue of the pregnant PG-treated cervix

Tissue samples were taken by means of a Silverman needle from the posterior lip of the cervix to a depth of 5–10 mm from 27 patients having an induced abortion between the 7th and 12th week of pregnancy. Eight hours prior to taking the sample 17 patients had an intracervical application of $PGF_{2\alpha}$ gel. The tissue samples were dried at $50\,^{\circ}C$; after hydrolysis amino acids were evaluated by means of an amino acid analyzer. Three amino acid analyses were made on each sample, and the mean values calculated for the amount of hydroxyproline residues per 1000 amino acid units of the collagen part of the total protein.

Quantitative amino acid analyses from different tissue depths of the cervix showed no significant differences regarding the amount of hydroxyproline. The distribution of individual hydroxyproline values showed a large variation in both groups; however, there was quite clearly a tendency to lower values, indicative of collagen loss, in the PG-treated as compared to the non-treated group (Fig. 5.5). There was also a lower value in the collagen fraction of total protein from nearly 80 % in the non-treated as compared to 68.6 % in the PG-treated cases.

The significance of this difference is made clear by the hydroxyproline distribution function (Fig. 5.6), which reflects the cumulative frequencies in

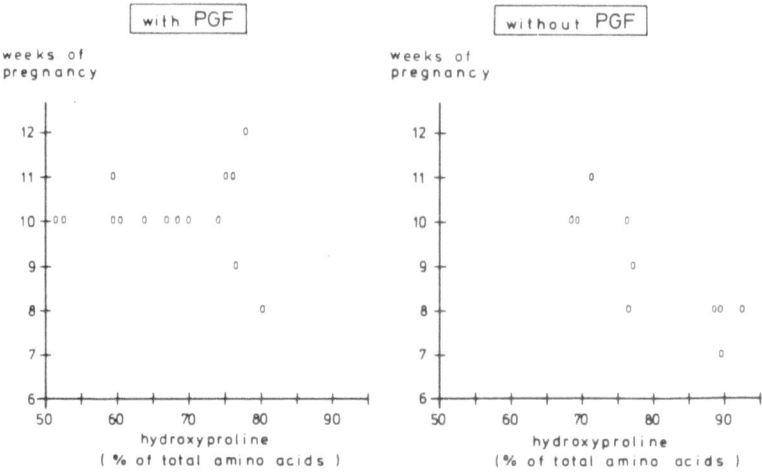

Figure 5.5 Individual hydroxyproline values and their correlation with weeks of pregnancy

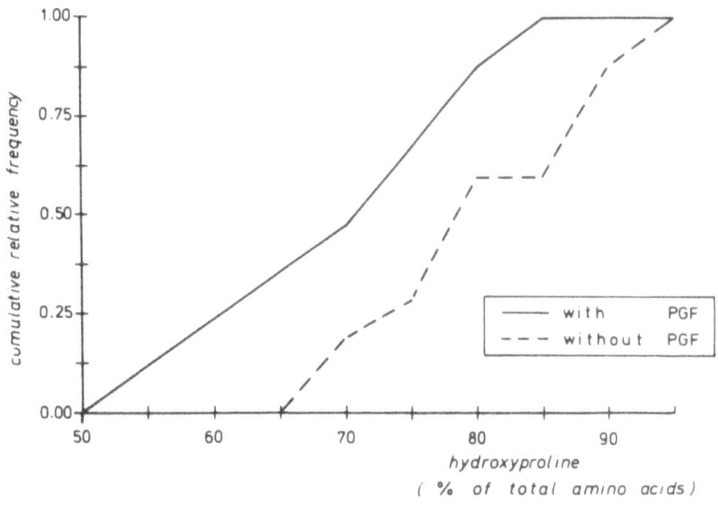

Figure 5.6 Hydroxyproline distribution function (with and without PG treatment)

the individual collectives; i.e. for each value on the abscissa the number of tissue samples with a hydroxyproline content equal to or less than this value is given. Lower hydroxyproline values were generally found in the PG-treated tissue samples; 50 % of them having a hydroxyproline content below 70 %, the figure being only 20 % in the untreated group. The significance of this difference was confirmed by a Wilcoxon test ($p = 0.016$).

A further decrease in collagen might be expected by increasing the time in which the PG gel is allowed to act on the cervix.

The average value of 80% for the collagen of the cervix during early pregnancy is rather similar to that of 82% reported by Danforth *et al.* (1974) for the non-pregnant cervix.

In contrast to our findings, Uldbjerg *et al.* (1981) found no significant changes in the total amount of collagen, estimated by the amount of hydroxyproline, whereas the concentration of sulfated glycosaminoglycans increased by almost 15%, 15 h after intracervical PGE_2 gel application.

Previous *in vitro* studies have confirmed the stimulating effect of $PGF_{2\alpha}$ on the production of glycosaminoglycans (Murota *et al.*, 1977). Data obtained from experiments of PG action on tissue components suggested that PG may alter glycosaminoglycans–collagen interactions that do not result in increasing collagen dissolution, but do result in a spacing or separation of collagen (Hillier and Wallis, 1981).

According to Norström (1982) PGs appear to have an inverse influence on the synthesis of collagen and proteoglycans, indicating an ability of the fibroblasts to adapt its metabolism in favor of either collagens or ground substance constituents.

The role of PGs in stimulating collagenase production is questionable. Although PGE_2 has been reported to stimulate macrophage collagenase production (Wahl *et al.*, 1979), no significant effect of either PGE_2 or $PGF_{2\alpha}$ has been found on active collagenase production by cervical tissue explants from late-pregnant or parturient ewes (Ellwood, 1981).

On the other hand, biological assays used to determine collagenolytic activities in cervical tissue of patients receiving locally applied PGE_2 demonstrated a significant rise in collagenolytic activity after local PG treatment (Szalay *et al.*, 1981).

These contradictory results clearly show that further investigations are necessary to clarify the mode of action of PGs on the cervix.

SUMMARY AND CONCLUSIONS

The intracervical application of PG gel has proved to be an efficient and safe method either for softening and dilating the cervix prior to surgical evacuation of the uterus in first trimester abortions or for treatment of the unfavorable cervix before induction of labor at term. The dilating effect of locally applied PG gel has been demonstrated objectively by tonometric methods. PG-induced ripening of the cervix appears to be independent of prominent uterine contractions, suggesting a direct effect of PG on the cervical connective tissue.

The histological appearance of the PG-treated cervix of early pregnancy shows the same changes as found in the pregnant cervix at term. The splitting and break-up of the collagen fibrils associated with the presence of cleavage products – verified by electron microscopy – support the theory of collagen breakdown. After PG pretreatment of the cervix a significant reduction in the collagen content such as occurs at term was observed, while the concentration of glycosaminoglycans appears to be increased.

These findings suggest that locally administered PG brings about ripening and dilatation of the cervix in a physiological manner. However, the mechanism of action of PG on the uterine cervix is still unknown. Attention has to be focused on the interrelationship between PG and the biosynthetic activity in the fibroblasts. In accordance with other workers we assume that PGs may have a role as modulators accelerating or reinforcing the current cellular metabolic activity in the fibroblast.

With respect to our current investigations it is hypothesized that PG may influence cellular protein phosphorylation by increasing calcium influx into the cells, and thus activating or inhibiting the adenylcyclase system. Further investigations are obviously necessary to establish this theory.

References

Berwind, T. (1954). Elektronenmikroskopische Untersuchungen am Fasersystem der Cervix uteri der Frau. *Arch. Gynecol.*, **184**, 459–468

Bryant, W. M., Greenwell, J. E. and Weeks, P. M. (1968). Alterations in collagen organization during dilatation of the cervix uteri. *Surg. Gynecol. Obstet.*, **126**, 27–39

Buckingham, J. C., Seldon, R. and Danforth, D. N. (1962). Connective tissue changes in the cervix during pregnancy and labor. *Ann. NY. Acad. Sci.*, **97**, 733–742

Bygdeman, M., Kwon, S. U., Mukherje, T. and Wiqvist, N. (1968). Effect of intravenous infusion of prostaglandin E_1 and E_2 on motility of the pregnant human uterus. *Am. J. Obstet. Gynecol.*, **102**, 317–326

Cabrol, D., Huszar, G., Romero, R. and Naftolin, F. (1981). Gestational changes in the rat uterine cervix: protein, collagen and glycosaminoglycans content. In Ellwood, D. A. and Anderson, A. B. M. (eds.) *The Cervix in Pregnancy and Labour*. pp. 34–39. (Edinburgh/London/Melbourne/New York: Churchill Livingstone)

Calder, A. A. (1981). The human cervix in pregnancy: a clinical perspective. In Ellwood, D. A. and Anderson, A. B. M. (eds.) *The Cervix in Pregnancy and Labour*. pp. 103–122. (Edinburgh/London/Melbourne/New York: Churchill Livingstone)

Conrad, J. T. and Ueland, K. (1976). Reduction of the stretch modulus of human cervical tissue by prostaglandin E_2. *Am. J. Obstet. Gynecol.*, **126**, 218–223

Danforth, D. N., Buckingham, J. C. and Roddick, J. W. (1960). Connective tissue changes incident to cervical effacement. *Am. J. Obstet. Gynecol.*, **80**, 939–945

Danforth, D. N., Veis, A., Breen, M., Weinstein, H. G., Buckingham, J. C. and Manalo, J. (1974). The effect of pregnancy and labor on the human cervix: changes in collagen, glycoproteins and glycosaminoglycans. *Am. J. Obstet. Gynecol.*, **120**, 641–651

Dingfelder, J. R., Brenner, W. E., Hendricks, C. H. and Staurovsky, L. G. (1975). Reduction of cervical resistance by prostaglandin suppositories prior to dilatation for induced abortion. *Am. J. Obstet. Gynecol.*, **122**, 25–30

Ellwood, D. A. (1981). The hormonal control of connective-tissue changes in the uterine cervix in pregnancy and at parturition. *Biochem. Soc. Trans.*, **8**, 662–667

Fitzpatrick, R. J. (1977). Dilatation of the uterine cervix. *Ciba Found. Symp.*, **47**, 31–39

Golichowski, A. (1980). Cervical stroma interstitial polysaccharide metabolism in pregnancy. In Naftolin, F. and Stubblefield, P. G. (eds.) *Dilatation of the Uterine Cervix*. pp. 99–112 (New York: Raven Press)

Harkness, M. L. R. and Harkness, R. D. (1959). Changes in the physical properties of the uterine cervix of the rat during pregnancy. *J. Physiol.*, **148**, 524–547

Haspels, A. A. and Neth, F. (1973). Induction of abortion by (1) intravenous and (2) intrauterine administration of $PGF_{2\alpha}$ (extra- and intraamniotic). *Adv. Biosci.*, **9**, 515–524

Hillier, K. and Wallis, R. M. (1981). Prostaglandins, steroids and the human cervix. In Ellwood, D. A. and Anderson, A. B. M. (eds.) *The Human Cervix in Pregnancy and Labour*. pp. 144–162. (Edinburgh/London/Melbourne/New York: Churchill Livingstone)

Hollingsworth, M. (1981). Softening of the rat cervix during pregnancy. In Ellwood, D. A. and

Anderson, A. B. M. (eds.) *The Human Cervix in Pregnancy and Labour.* pp. 13–33. (Edinburgh/London/Melbourne/New York: Churchill Livingstone)

Hulka, J. F., Lefler, H. T., Angelone, H. and Lachenbruch, P. A. (1974). A new electronic force monitor to measure factors influencing cervical dilatation for vacuum curettage. *Am. J. Obstet. Gynecol.,* **120,** 166–173

Junquira, L. C. U., Zugaib, M., Montes, G. S., Toledo, O. M. S., Krisztan, R. M. and Shigihara, K. M. (1980). Morphologic and histochemical evidence for the occurrence of collagenolysis and for the role of neutrophilic polymorpho nuclear leucocytes during cervical dilatation. *Am. J. Obstet. Gynecol.,* **138,** 273–281

Karim, S. M. M., Trussel, R. R., Patel, R. C. and Hillier, K. (1968). Response of pregnant human uterus to prostaglandin $F_{2\alpha}$ induction of labor. *Br. Med. J.,* **4,** 621–623

Karim, S. M. M., Ng, S. C. and Ratnam, S. S. (1979). Termination of abnormal intrauterine pregnancy with prostaglandins. In Karim, S. M. M. (ed.) *Advances in Prostaglandins Research, Practical Application of Prostaglandins and their Synthesis Inhibitors.* pp. 319–374. (Lancaster: MTP Press)

Kleissl, H. P., van der Rest, M., Naftolin, F., Glorieux, F. H. and De Leon, A. (1978). Collagen changes in the human uterine cervix at parturition. *Am. J. Obstet. Gynecol.,* **130,** 748–753

Kühnle, H., Grande, P. and Kuhn, W. (1977). Preventing complications due to dilatation by intracervical application of a prostaglandin gel. *Geburtsh. u. Frauenheilk.,* **37,** 675–680

Liggins, G. C. (1978). Ripening of the cervix. *Sem. Perinat.,* **2,** 261–271

Lippert, T. H. (1979). The use of prostaglandin gel in obstetrics and gynecology. *Arch. Gynecol.,* **227,** 171–179

Lippert, T. H., Fridrich, S., Schneider, H. P. and Briel, R. C. (1982). Über die Beeinflussung der Dehnbarkeit der Rattenzervix durch die Prostaglandine E_2 und $F_{2\alpha}$. *44. Tag Dtsch. Ges. f. Gyn. u. Geburtsh. München, 13.9.–17.9.1982,* Abstract 138

Liu, D. T. Y., Black, M. M., Melcher, D. H., Melville, H. A. H., Cameron, S. and Morgan, J. (1975). Dilatation of the parous non-pregnant cervix. *Br. J. Obstet. Gynaecol.,* **82,** 246–251

MacKenzie, J. Z. (1981). Clinical studies on cervical ripening. In Ellwood, D. A. and Anderson, A. B. M. (eds.) *The Human Cervix in Pregnancy and Labour.* pp. 163–186. (Edinburgh/London/Melbourne/New York: Churchill Livingstone)

MacKenzie, J. Z. and Embrey, M. P. (1979). A comparison of PGE_2 and $PGF_{2\alpha}$ vaginal gel for ripening the cervix before induction of labour. *Br. J. Obstet. Gynaecol.,* **86,** 167–170

Maillot, K. V., Stuhlsatz, H. W., Mohanaradhakrishnan, V. and Greiling, H. (1979). Changes in the glycosaminoglycans distribution pattern in the human uterine cervix during pregnancy and labor. *Am. J. Obstet. Gynecol.,* **135,** 503–506

Maillot, K. V., Stuhlsatz, H. W. and Gentsch, H. H. (1981). Connective tissue changes in the human cervix in pregnancy and labour. In Ellwood, D. A. and Anderson, A. B. M. (eds.). *The Human Cervix in Pregnancy and Labour.* pp. 123–135. (Edinburgh/London/Melbourne/New York: Churchill Livingstone)

Mori, Y., Ito, A., Hirakawa, S. and Kitamura, K. (1981). Proteinases in the human and rabbit cervix. In Ellwood, D. A. and Anderson, A. B. M. (eds.) *The Human Cervix in Pregnancy and Labour.* pp. 136–143. (Edinburgh/London/Melbourne/New York: Churchill Livingstone)

Murota, S., Abe, M. and Otsuka, K. (1977). Stimulatory effect of prostaglandins on the production of hexosamine-containing substances by cultured fibroblasts (3). Induction of hyaluronic acid synthetase by prostaglandin $F_{2\alpha}$ *Prostaglandins,* **14,** 983–991

Norström, A. (1982). Influence of prostaglandin E_2 on the biosynthesis of connective tissue constituents in the pregnant human cervix. *Prostaglandins,* **23,** 361–367

Norström, A., Wilhelmsson, L. and Hamberger, K. (1981). The regulatory influence of prostaglandins on protein synthesis in the human non-pregnant cervix. *Prostaglandins,* **22,** 117–124

Parry, Dilys, M. and Ellwood, D. A. (1981). Ultrastructural aspects of cervical softening in the sheep. In Ellwood, D. A. and Anderson, A. B. M. (eds.) *The Human Cervix in Pregnancy and Labour.* pp. 74–84. (Edinburgh/London/Melbourne/New York: Churchill Livingstone)

Rath, W., Kühnle, H., Theobald, P. and Kuhn, W. (1982). Objective demonstration of cervical softening with a prostaglandin $F_{2\alpha}$ gel during first trimester abortion. *Int. J. Gynaecol. Obstet.,* **20,** 195–199

Saito, Y., Takahashi, S. and Maki, M. (1981). Effects of some drugs on ripening of uterine cervix in non-pregnant castrated and pregnant rats. *Tohoku J. Exp. Med.,* **133,** 205–220

Steiner, H., Zahradnik, H. P., Breckwoldt, M., Robrecht, D. and Hillemanns, H. G. (1979). Cervical ripening prior to induction of labour (intracervical application of PGE_2 viscous gel). *Prostaglandins*, **17**, 125–133

Stys, S. J., Clewell, W. H. and Meschia, G. (1978). Changes in cervical compliance at parturition independent of uterine activity. *Am. J. Obstet. Gynecol.*, **130**, 414–418

Szalay, S., Husslein, P. and Grünberger, W. (1981). Collagenolytic activity of human cervical tissue, following local application of prostaglandin E_2 (PGE_2) using a portio adapter. *Zbl. Gynäkol.*, **103**, 1107–1112

Takahashi, S., Saito, Y., Taguchi, J. and Maki, M. (1978). Scanning electron microscopic study on the effects of prostaglandin E_2, dehydroepiandrosterone sulfate, relaxin and oxytocin on connective tissue of uterine cervix of late-pregnant rat. *J. Clin. Electron. Microscopy*, **11**, 730

Toppozada, M., Bygdeman, M., Papageorgiou, C. and Wiqvist, N. (1973). Administration of 15me-$PGF_{2\alpha}$ as a pre-operative means of cervical dilatation. *Prostaglandins*, **4**, 371–379

Uldbjerg, N., Ekman, G., Malmström. A., Sporrong, B., Ulmsten, U. and Wingerup, L. (1981). Biochemical and morphological changes of human cervix after local application of prostaglandin E_2 in pregnancy. *Lancet*, **1**, 267–268

Ulmsten, U. (1979). Aspects on ripening of the cervix and induction of labor by intracervical application of PGE_2 in viscous gel. *Acta Obstet. Gynecol. Scand.*, Suppl. **84**, 5–9

Ulmsten, U. and Wingerup, L. (1980). Clinical experiences with a new gel for intracervical application of prostaglandin E_2 before therapeutic abortion or induction of term labor. *Prostaglandins*, **20**, 533–546

Ulmsten, U., Kirstein-Pedersen, A., Stenberg, P. and Wingerup, L. (1979). A new gel for intracervical application of prostaglandin E_2. *Acta Obstet. Gynecol. Scand.*, Suppl. **84**, 19–21

Veis, A. (1980). Cervical dilatation: a proteolytic mechanism for loosening the collagen fiber network. In Naftolin, F. and Stubblefield, P. G. (eds.) *Dilatation of the Uterine Cervix*. pp. 192–202. (New York: Raven Press)

Wahl, L. M., Olsen, C. E., Wahl, S. M., Sandberg, A. L. and Morgenhagen, S. E. (1979). Prostaglandin-regulated macrophage collagenase. In Horton, J. E., Torpley, T. M. and Davies, W. F. (eds.). *Mechanism of Localised Bone Loss*. Special supplement to calcified tissue abstracts. pp. 181–190. Information Retrieval Inc.

Wingerup, L., Ulmsten, U. and Andersson, K.-E. (1979). Ripening of the cervix by intracervical application of PGE_2 gel before termination of pregnancy with dilatation and evacuation. *Acta Obstet. Gynaecol. Scand.*, Suppl. **84**, 15–18

6
Interaction between prostaglandins and catecholamines on cervical collagen

L. WILHELMSSON, A. NORSTRÖM, J. TJUGUM and L. HAMBERGER

INTRODUCTION

The human cervix can today be considered as a separate functional entity within the uterus in comparison with an earlier widespread opinion that this structure merely played a passive role secondarily to contractions of the uterine body. This new view is based upon investigations demonstrating that hormones and prostaglandins are able to interfere with cervical connective tissue independently of myometrial activity (Schild *et al.*, 1951; Novy and Liggins, 1980). Thus, prostaglandins of both E- and F-series have been shown, in clinical studies, to act on the cervix apart from their effect on the myometrium (MacLennan and Green, 1979; Ulmsten, 1979; Forman *et al.*, 1982). From these and other studies from our laboratory (Norström *et al.*, 1981; Norström, 1982), it seems reasonable to suggest that PGs act directly on the fibrous connective tissue, which constitutes the major part of the cervix (Danforth, 1974; Hughesdon, 1952).

The upper portion of the human cervix is innervated by short adrenergic neurons originating in peripheral ganglion formations at the uterovaginal junction (Owman *et al.*, 1974). These specific sympathetic nerves are partly characterized by alterations in their noradrenalin content during pregnancy (Sjöberg, 1968; Owman *et al.*, 1975). Likewise, tissue fluctuations in noradrenalin content during non-pregnant conditions could be related to the actual state of the sexual steroids (Thorbert, 1978). Further, various PGs of the E-series have been reported to modulate the autonomic nervous system in different organs (Hedqvist, 1970; Brody and Kadowitz, 1974).

All these former studies indicate that PGs and catecholamines can exert an intermingled action on cervical tissue. This series of experiments was therefore designed to investigate the interaction between PGs and catecholamines on cervical collagen biosynthesis in pregnant, as well as in non-pregnant, women under different hormonal conditions.

MATERIAL AND METHODS

Cervical tissue was obtained from fertile non-pregnant women undergoing hysterectomy due to a benign gynecological disease. Immediately after removal of the uterus cervical blocks were excised from the fibrous inner portion of the upper cervix. These blocks were mechanically chopped into 1 mm thick slices (wet weight 5–10 mg) (see Norström et al., 1981). Tissue from pregnant women was taken both as needle biopsies from the cervix and as excisions from the lower uterine segment in subjects undergoing cesarean section (see Norström, 1982).

The specimens obtained were preincubated in Krebs Ringer bicarbonate buffer (KRB) (10 ml Ehrlenmeyer flasks) fortified with PGE_2 and noradrenalin (NA) in various combinations. Upon preincubation (60 min) the pieces were transferred to fresh buffer containing [^{3}H]proline together with the above-mentioned compounds and incubated for another 60 min at 37°C in a gas atmosphere of 5 % CO_2 in oxygen. Incubation was terminated by washing the specimens in chilled buffer containing unlabelled proline (1 μM). In one experimental series the specimens were blotted on filter paper and homogenized in 5 % perchloroacetic acid. After centrifugation samples were taken for determination of radioactivity in a Packard liquid scintillation counter (model 2450, Tri Carb). The protein content was determined according to Lowry et al. (1951). In another series of experiments the tissue pieces were incubated in 12 % (w/v) trichloracetic acid and washed twice in a chloroform–methanol mixture (2:1). After drying in an oven for a period of 24 h the remaining dry material was weighed using a Cahn microbalance (model 4700) and then dissolved in 0.25 ml Soluene® (Packard Company, USA). Further methodological details are given elsewhere (Norström et al., 1981).

Chemicals and Hormones

[^{3}H]Proline (0.25 mCi/μmol; 0.2 mmol) (NEN-Chemicals, USA); noradrenalin bitartrate (Noradrenalin, Apoteks-bolaget, Sweden); PGE_2, crystalline sodium salt (Upjohn, Co., USA), dissolved in 99.5 % ethanol to obtain stock solutions, further diluted in buffer before each experiment; reserpine (Serpasil, CIBA, USA).

RESULTS

Cervical specimens obtained from patients being in the late follicular phase were incubated for 60 min in the presence of noradrenalin (1 μg/ml) and the incorporation of [^{3}H]proline into total protein determined. This treatment caused a significant increase of the net incorporation, an effect which could be effectively blocked by concomitant presence of PGE_2 (Fig. 6.1).

In specimens obtained in the early luteal phase [^{3}H]proline incorporation was incubated by noradrenalin as compared with control specimens. Concomitant presence of noradrenalin and PGE_2 in the incubation medium turned the inhibitory effect by noradrenalin alone into a stimulation (Fig. 6.2).

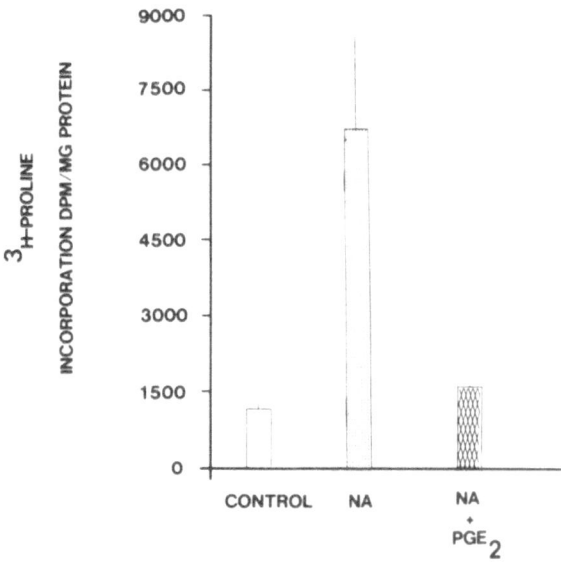

Figure 6.1 Effects of NA (1 μg/ml) and PGE$_2$ (300 ng/ml) on the incorporation of [^{3}H]proline in cervical tissue specimens in the late follicular phase. Note the counteraction of PGE$_2$ on the NA-induced increase of [^{3}H]proline labeling. (From Wilhelmsson *et al.*, 1982, by permission)

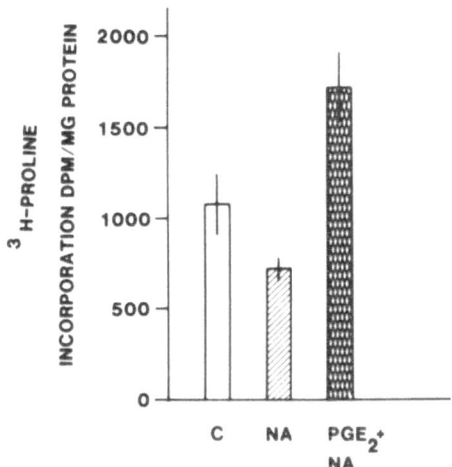

Figure 6.2 Preparations from the luteal phase, incubated in the presence of NA (1 μg/ml) and PGE$_2$ (300 ng/ml). PGE$_2$ counteracts the inhibitory effect of NA. (From Wilhelmsson *et al.*, 1982, by permission)

Pregnant cervical tissue

Specimens obtained during the first trimester responded to noradrenalin *in vitro* with a pronounced reduction of [^{3}H]proline incorporation (Fig. 6.3).

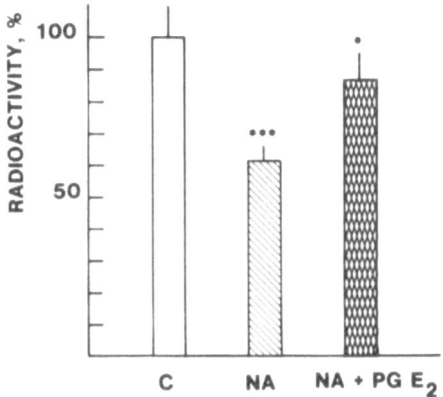

Figure 6.3 Incubation of cervical specimens from women during the first trimester of pregnancy. The inhibition of [³H]proline incorporation of NA (1 μg/ml) is effectively counteracted by PGE₂ (300 ng/ml). (From Norstrom *et al.*, to be published)

This inhibition of [³H]proline incorporation into total protein could be effectively counteracted by PGE₂.

In specimens obtained from patients close to term [³H]proline incorporation was still inhibited by noradrenalin (Fig. 6.4) while no influence by concomitant presence of PGE₂ was obtained.

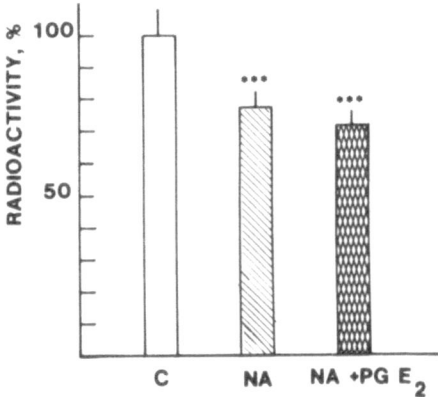

Figure 6.4 NA (1 μg/ml) reduced the [³H]proline labeling in tissue from the lower uterine segment at term pregnancy. At this stage PGE₂ (300 ng/ml) did not significantly interfere with the action of NA. (From Norstrom *et al.*, to be published)

DISCUSSION

In previous studies from this laboratory evidence has been gained in favor of the view that the incorporation of [³H]proline into total protein is representative for the collagen net synthesis in cervical tissue. It is suggested that protein incorporation appears to reflect cervical plasticity in a more adequate manner than static determinations of collagen content. In accordance with the clinically well-documented role of PGs in the process of cervical softening and ripening various PGs have been shown to possess a regulatory influence upon collagen net synthesis *in vitro* (Norström *et al.*,1981; Norström, 1982)

The present results show that not only PGs, but also the neurotransmitters, modulate the net collagen synthesis and, hence, cervical maturation. The very existence of smooth muscle in the cervix has led to the conclusion that the sympathetic nerves are merely attached to smooth muscle function. However, the data presented demonstrate that noradrenalin may also interfere with cervical collagen metabolism. A proposed sphincter-like function in the cervix is therefore not only based upon the musculature but also the connective tissue seems to be involved. Both PGs and catecholamines have probably a regulatory influence upon this sphincter mechanism. The difference in response in specimens from non-pregnant and pregnant patients, as well as in specimens obtained from various phases of the cycle, indicate that steroids may also be of importance in this connection. This effect may be induced by a direct action of sex steroids on the cervical tissue but may also be due to a hormonally induced alteration in the tissue contents of PGs and catecholamines.

Acknowledgements

The present work was supported by grants from Tore Nilsson's Foundation, Harald and Greata Jeansson's Foundation and 'Expressen' Prenatal Research Foundation.

References

Brody, M. J. and Kadowitz, P. J. (1974). Prostaglandins as modulators of the anatomic nervous system. *Fed. Proc.*, **33**, 48–60

Danforth, D. N. (1974). The fibrous nature of the human cervix, and its relation to the isthmic segment in gravid and nongravid uteri. *Am. J. Obstet. Gynecol.*, **53**, 541–560

Forman, A., Ulmsten, U., Bányai, J., Wingerup, L. and Uldbjerg, N. (1982). Evidence for a local effect of intracervical prostaglandin E_2-gel. *Am. J. Obstet. Gynecol.*, **143**, 756–760

Hedqvist, P. (1970). Studies on the effect of prostaglandin E_1 and E_2 in the sympathetic neuromuscular transmission in some animal tissues. *Acta Physiol. Scand.*, Suppl. **345**, p.1

Hughesdon, M. K. (1952). The fibromuscular structure of the cervix and its changes during pregnancy and labour. *J. Obstet. Gynecol. Br. Emp.*, **59**, 763–776

Lowry, O. H., Rosebrough, R., Farr, A. L. and Randall, J. (1951). Protein measurement with the folin phenol reagent. *J. Biol. Chem.*, **193**, 265–275

MacLennan, A. H. and Green, R. C. (1979). Cervical ripening and induction of labour with intravaginal prostaglandin $F_{2\alpha}$. *Lancet*, **1**, 117–119

Norström, A. (1982). Influence of prostaglandin E_2 on the biosynthesis of connective tissue constituents on the pregnant human cervix. *Prostaglandins*, **23**, 361–368

Norström, A., Wilhelmsson, L. and Hamberger, L. (1981). The regulatory influence of prostaglandin on protein synthesis in the human non-pregnant cervix. *Prostaglandins*, **22**, 117–123

Novy, M. J. and Liggins, G. C. (1980). Role of prostaglandins, prostacyclin and thromboxane in the physiological control of the uterus and in parturition. *Semin. Perinat.*, **4**, 45–66

Owman, Ch., Sjöberg, N. O. and Sjöstrand, N. O. (1974). Short adrenergic neurons, a peripheral neuro-endocrine mechanism, In Fujwara, M. and Tanaka, C. (eds.) *Amino Fluorescence Histochemistry.* pp. 47–66. (Tokyo: Igaku Shoin)

Owman, Ch., Alm., P., Rosengren, E., Sjöberg, N. O. and Thorbert, G. (1975). Variation in the level of uterine norepinephrine during pregnancy in the guinea pig. *Am J. Obstet. Gynecol.,* **122,** 961–964

Schild, H. O., Fitzpatrick, R. J. and Nixon, W. C. W. (1951). Activity of the human cervix and corpus uteri. *Lancet,* **260,** 250–253

Sjöberg, N. O. (1968). Considerations on the cause of disappearance of the adrenergic transmitter in uterine nerves during pregnancy. *Acta Physiol. Scand.,* **72,** 510–517

Thorbert, G. (1978). Regional changes in structure and function of adrenergic nerves in guinea pig uterus during pregnancy. *Acta Obstet. Gynecol. Scand.,* Suppl. **79,** p.000

Ulmsten, U. (1979). Aspects on ripening of the cervix and induction of labour by intracervical application of PGE_2 in viscous gel. *Acta Obstet. Gynecol. Scand.,* Suppl. **184,** pp. 5–9

Section II
Clinical Applications

7
Self-administration at home of prostaglandin for termination of early pregnancy

M. BYGDEMAN, N. J. CHRISTENSEN, K. GRÉEN and O. VESTERQVIST

INTRODUCTION

The possibility of using prostaglandins for termination of early pregnancy was evaluated in 1971 (Karim, 1971). One of the objectives has been to develop a non-surgical, out-patient, possibly self-administered method as an alternative to vacuum aspiration in very early pregnancy (up to 49 days of amenorrhea).

The experience of vaginal administration of natural prostaglandins for termination of early pregnancy has, in general, been discouraging. Effective dose schedules are associated with a high frequency of gastrointestinal side-effects (Tredway and Mishell, 1973). Intrauterine administration seems to be the only method with a predictable uterine response and a high efficacy if PGE_2 or $PGF_{2\alpha}$ were used. To reduce side-effects to an acceptable level, however, premedication is still necessary (Mocsary and Csapo, 1975). New prostaglandin analogs have continuously been developed and tested clinically (Karim et al., 1977; Bygdeman et al., 1979, 1980; Takagi et al., 1978). The latest generation of E-analogs seems to be significantly superior to those evaluated previously. It therefore seemed appropriate to study whether self-treatment at home was a possibility using vaginal suppositories containing one of the new stable E-analogs, 9-deoxo-16,16-dimethyl-9-methylene PGE_2 (9-methylene PGE_2) (Bygdeman et al., 1979; Kimball et al., 1979). We have earlier reported on the first 40 treated patients (Bygdeman et al., 1981).

PATIENTS AND METHODS

Altogether 100 patients agreed to treat themselves at home. The patients were selected from those coming to the hospital for an early therapeutic abortion. The selection criteria were a healthy patient, a normal pregnancy (judged by gynecological examination and plasma-HCG), an amenorrhea of up to 49 days, at least one previous pregnancy, and that the patient accepted a non-

Table 7.1 Composition of the suppositories. Amount of active substance in a base consisting of a mixture of Witepsol H-15 and Witepsol E-76

Amount of 9-methylene PGE$_2$	Amount of H-15/E-76 (1:4) in each suppository	No. of patients
75 mg + 30 mg	2.2 g	48
60 mg + 45 mg	2.2 g/1.7 g	16
50 mg × 2	1.8 g	15
60 mg × 2	2.2 g	13
60 mg × 2	1.8 g	8
		100

surgical procedure would be used. The patient's mean age was 33.5 years, number of previous pregnancies 3.9, and parity 2.0. Duration of amenorrhea was, as a mean, 44.3 days (range 39–49 days).

Each patient fulfilling the criteria mentioned above obtained two suppositories both containing 9-methylene PGE$_2$ as the active uterotonic drug, but dispensed in different amounts of a triglyceride base consisting of a mixture of Witepsol H-15 and E-76 (1:.4) (Dynamite-Nobel AG, Witten, West Germany) as showed in Table 7.1. The total amount of drug given to the patients varied between 100 and 120 mg, resulting in a plasma level between 10 and 30 ng/ml for approximately 10 h (Figs 7.1 and 7.2) (Gréen et al., 1982). Since the results were similar for all treatment groups, the outcome of therapy, side-effects and complications were calculated for all patients as one group.

The patients placed the vaginal suppositories as far up in the vagina as possible at a 6-h interval. In most cases the treatment started in the evening.

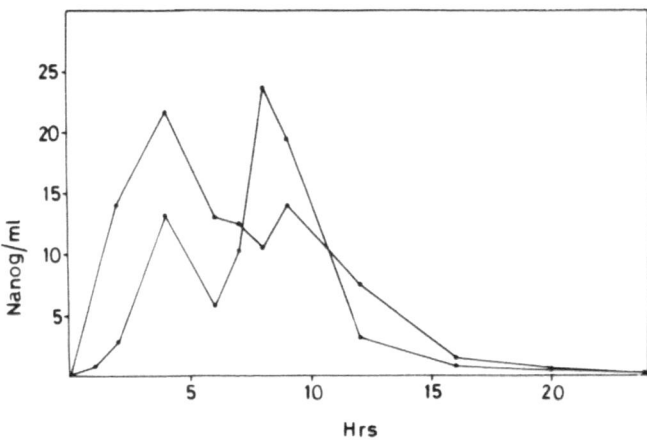

Figure 7.1 Plasma levels of 9-methylene PGE$_2$ following vaginal administration of 50 mg followed by 50 mg 6 h later. The concentration of the analog was measured by gas chromatography–mass spectrometry (Green et al., 1982)

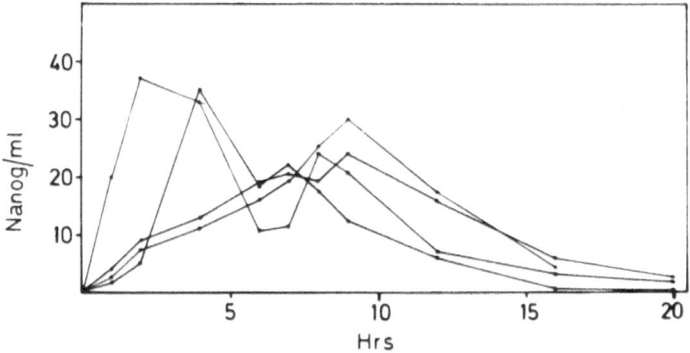

Figure 7.2 Plasma levels of 9-methylene PGE$_2$ following vaginal administration of 60 mg followed by 45 mg 6 h later. The concentration of the analog was measured by gas chromatography–mass spectrometry (Green *et al.*, 1982)

One member of the research staff was always available at the hospital to allow the patient to call if anything unexpected happened. Each patient carefully recorded side-effects, temperature, start, duration and the amount of bleeding and appearance of the first menstrual period after treatment.

All patients attended two follow-up visits, 1 and 2 weeks after treatment. At the follow-up visits, hemoglobin value and plasma β-HCG was measured, and at the second visit a gynecological examination was performed. At the second follow-up visit the outcome of therapy was first judged as a complete abortion (rapid or delayed expulsion) or a continuation of the pregnancy. The judgment was based on the duration and amount of bleeding, pattern of plasma β-HCG decrease, gynecological examination, and if no obvious signs were present that the patient had aborted completely, ultrasound examination. If clinically indicated, additional follow-up visits were scheduled. If curettage was necessary during the time from the second follow-up visit to the first menstruation, the outcome of the therapy was based on the histopathological examination. The time for the first menstruation and its characteristics were reported by the patient by answering a number of relevant questions on a special form sent in by post.

RESULTS

Altogether 100 early pregnant patients agreed to use a non-surgical abortion method and to treat themselves at home. In 94% of the patients the therapy was regarded as successful (complete abortion). In the majority of the patients ($n = 89$) plasma β-HCG rapidly decreased and was less than 1500 IU/l 2 weeks after the start of treatment, indicating an expulsion of the conceptus during or shortly after treatment. In the remaining five patients with a complete abortion at least part of the conceptus remained in the uterus for a longer time if judged from the slower decrease in plasma β-

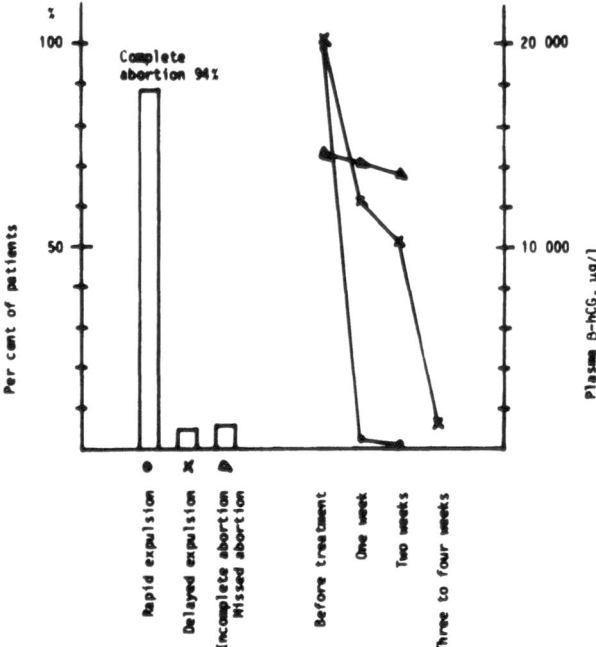

Figure 7.3 Outcome of therapy following treatment with 9-methylene PGE$_2$ at home. The patients were divided into three groups depending on the decrease rate of plasma β-HCG

HCG levels. In none of these 94 patients was a surgical intervention necessary. In the six unsuccessfully treated patients the plasma HCG level remained unchanged and the ultrasound examination prior to curettage and the histopathological examination of the conceptus indicated a missed abortion (Fig. 7.3).

The treatment resulted in an increased uterine contractility followed by vaginal bleeding in all patients. The bleeding started as a rule 3–6 h after the start of treatment. The duration of bleeding was 9–14 days in the majority of patients (Table 7.2). The patients who did not abort had a tendency to start bleeding later, and to bleed for a shorter time, than the patients judged as complete abortion. The hemoglobin value did not change significantly during the 2 weeks observation period in any of the patients.

Table 7.2 Bleeding pattern: mean values and (range)

Clinical course	Start of bleeding (hours)	Duration of bleeding (days)	No. of patients
Complete abortion			
Rapid decrease in β-HCG	3.9 (1–12)	11.4 (3–22)	$n = 89$
Slow decrease in β-HCG	4.6 (2–12)	8.6 (2–18)	$n = 5$
Missed abortion	7 (2–14)	5 (1–12)	$n = 6$

Forty-five patients (45 %) had no side-effects. Almost 40 % of the patients experienced occasional episodes of vomiting and/or diarrhea (Fig. 7.4). In 66 patients (66 %) the treatment was associated with no, or only slight, pain. Four women found the uterine pain unacceptable (4 %) and called the hospital 3–4 h after the start of therapy for assistance. The patients were admitted to the hospital and received one intramuscular injection of meperidine chloride, which was sufficient to alleviate the pain. Thirty patients (30 %) experienced moderate uterine pain, which could be alleviated at home with one suppository of 50 mg pentazocine (Fortalgesic®). A temperature elevation of more than 38 °C was observed in 25 % of the patients, and in 4 % of the patients the temperature exceeded 39 °C. The temperature returned to normal within a few hours after the insertion of the last suppository. The first menstrual period appeared as a mean after 35 days (range 25–48 days) and did not differ significantly from the patients' normal periods.

Two patients (2 %) had clinical signs of endometritis, mainly subjective pain and pain at the gynecological examination. Neither of these two patients showed temperature rise, leukocytosis or increased erythrocyte sedimentation rate. The patients were successfully treated with tetracyclin for 1 week at home.

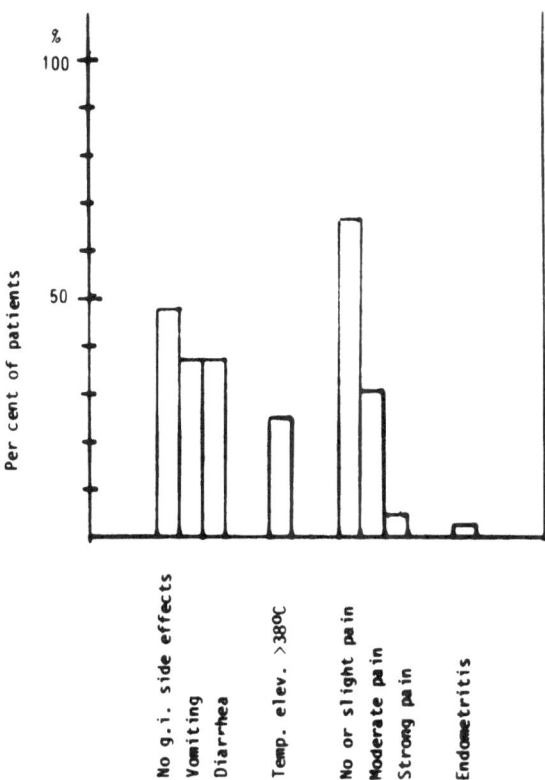

Figure 7.4 Side-effects and complications following vaginal administration of 9-methylene PGE$_2$ at home

DISCUSSION

Nearly 15 years ago it was shown that natural prostaglandins were effective in stimulating uterine contractility during all phases of pregnancy. Since then it has been hoped that a non-surgical self-administered alternative to vacuum aspiration for termination of early pregnancy could be developed. Natural prostaglandins proved, however, unsatisfactory in this respect.

New stable prostaglandin E-analogs suitable for vaginal administration or intramuscular injection have been developed during the few past years. Effective dose schedules were associated with a low frequency of gastrointestinal side-effects, significantly lower than that reported for previously available F-analogs (Bygdeman, 1979). One of the new E-analogs, 9-deoxo-16,16-dimethyl-9-methylene PGE_2, was used in the present investigation. Previous studies have indicated that this analog is at least comparable to the two other analogs evaluated, i.e. 16,16-dimethyl-trans-Δ^2-PGE_1 methyl ester and 16-phenoxy-ω-17,18,19,20-tetranor PGE_2 methyl sulfonylamide (Karim *et al.*, 1977; Takagi *et al.*, 1978; Bygdeman *et al.*, 1981, 1983).

In an earlier study vaginal suppositories containing 75 mg 9-deoxy-16,16-dimethyl-9-methylene PGE_2 given at 0 and 6 h resulted in a complete abortion in all patients ($n = 25$) treated during early pregnancy. The main problem associated with this treatment schedule was uterine pain, making parenteral administration of analgesics necessary in 35 % of the patients (Bygdeman *et al.*, 1980). In order to minimize the degree of pain, suppositories with a reduced amount of drug were used. Furthermore, only patients with a previous pregnancy, and thus aware of the nature of uterine contractions, were allowed to participate in the study.

The present study has shown that vaginal administration of 9-methylene PGE_2 was highly effective in terminating early pregnancy even if administered by the patient herself at home. Clinical course, gynecological examination and plasma β-HCG demonstrated a complete abortion in 94 % of the treated patients. It is noteworthy that in five of these patients the decrease in plasma β-HCG was relatively slow, but still the whole conceptus was eventually expelled without any complications. The conclusion is that even if plasma β-HCG 2 weeks after treatment has decreased to only 50 % of its initial value, it seems acceptable to delay surgical intervention if bleeding complications are not present. The lack of such an expectative attitude may be one explanation for the relatively low 'success rate' reported from some centers when using prostaglandins for termination of early pregnancy.

Gastrointestinal side-effects occurred in about 40 % of the 100 patients. In the patients who experienced these side-effects the frequency was limited to one or two episodes per patient. Only five of the home-treated patients regarded the degree of gastrointestinal side-effects as disturbingly high. The frequency was comparable to that previously reported for hospital treatment with the analog (Bygdeman *et al.*, 1980) and lower than that found for vaginal administration of F-analogs, e.g. 15-methyl $PGF_{2\alpha}$ methyl ester (Bygdeman, 1979).

For the acceptability of a self-administered method used by the women at home, the degree of pain associated with the treatment is of great importance.

In the present study only four of the patients needed analgesic injections for an effective alleviation of pain in comparison with 35 % in the pilot study when the higher dose was used (75 mg at 0 and 6 h) and the patients were treated in the hospital (Bygdeman *et al.*, 1980). It is likely that the low frequency of uterine pain was partly due to the reduced dose, but the different types of environment and the selection of patients might also have been of importance. Bleeding was also no problem. None of the patients experienced a heavy blood loss. The mean blood loss during the entire bleeding period has previously been found to be 61 ml (Bygdeman *et al.*, 1983).

The results of the present study indicate that termination of early pregnancy by self-treatment at home starts to be a reality, at least in selected patients. Almost all patients had a positive attitude to the treatment. The most common reasons were the anonymity of the therapy, the possibility of the husband to participate and the more 'natural' procedure as compared to vacuum aspiration.

Acknowledgements

We are grateful to the Upjohn Company, Kalamazoo, Michigan, USA, for supplying the drug, 9-deoxo-16,16-dimethyl-9-methylene PGE_2, and for financial support. Part of the study was also supported by a research grant from the Special Programme of Research, Development and Research Training of the World Health Organization.

References

Bygdeman, M. (1979). Menstrual regulation with prostaglandins. In Karim, S. M. M. (ed.). *Practical Applications of Prostaglandins and their Synthesis Inhibitors.* pp. 267–282. (Lancaster: MTP Press)

Bygdeman, M., Bremme, K., Christensen, N., Lundström, V. and Gréen, K. (1980). A comparison of two stable prostaglandin E analogues for termination of early pregnancy and for cervical dilatation. *Contraception*, 22, 471–483

Bygdeman, M., Christensen, N., Gréen, K. and Zheng, S. (1981). Self-administration of prostaglandin for termination of early pregnancy. *Contraception*, 24, 45–52

Bygdeman, M., Christensen, N. J., Gréen, K., Zheng, S. and Lundström, V. (1983). Termination of early pregnancy. Future development. *Acta Obstet. Gynecol. Scand.*, Suppl. 113, 125–129

Bygdeman, M., Gréen, K., Bergström, S., Bundy, G. and Kimball, F. (1979). New prostaglandin E_2 analogue for pregnancy termination. *Lancet*, 1, 1136

Gréen, K., Vesterqvist, O., Bygdeman, M., Christensen, N. J. and Bergström, S. (1982). Plasma levels of 9-deoxo-16,16-dimethyl-9-methylene PGE_2 in connection with its development as an abortifacient. *Prostaglandins*, 24, 451–466

Karim, S. M. M. (1971). Once-a-month vaginal administration of prostaglandins E_2 and $F_{2\alpha}$ for fertility control. *Contraception*, 3, 173–183

Karim, S. M. M., Rao, B., Ratnam, S. S., Prasad, R. N. V., Wong, Y. M. and Ilancheran, A. (1977). Termination of early pregnancy (menstrual induction) with 16-phenoxy-ω-tetrano PGE_2 methyl sulfonylamide. *Contraception*, 16, 377–381

Kimball, F. A., Bundy, G. L., Robert, A. and Weeks, J. R. (1979). Synthesis and biological properties of 9-deoxo-16,16-dimethyl-9-methylene PGE_2. *Prostaglandins*, 17, 657–666

Mocsary, P. and Csapo, A. I. (1975). Work in progress. Menstrual induction with $PGF_{2\alpha}$ and PGE_2. *Prostaglandins*, 10, 545–547

Takagi, S., Sakata, H., Yoshida, T., Den, K., Fujii, K., Amemiya, H. and Tomita, M. (1978). Termination of early pregnancy by ONO-802 suppositories (16,16-dimethyl-trans-Δ^2-PGE$_1$ methyl ester). *Prostaglandins*, **15**, 913–919

Tredway, D. R. and Mishell, D. R. (1973). Therapeutic abortion of early human gestation with vaginal suppositories of prostaglandin F$_{2\alpha}$. *Am. J. Obstet. Gynecol.*, **116**, 795–798

8
Menstrual induction and cervical priming prior to evacuation

N. H. LAUERSEN and Z. R. GRAVES

INTRODUCTION

As the number of reported induced abortions in the United States approaches one million, it becomes more important to develop effective abortion techniques, free of both immediate complications and sequelae. Early interruption techniques are particularly attractive since, as a general rule, the number of procedure-related complications increases as gestation lengthens. The demand for early interruption has been enhanced both by an increasingly informed patient population and the availability of highly sensitive pregnancy tests which are 95 % accurate within days after conception.

Many physicians are hesitant to terminate early pregnancies since some of the products of conception may be retained. For this reason, patients are often asked to wait until 8 weeks of gestation, although prolonging the pregnancy may cause psychological and physiological hardship. Two methods of facilitating early pregnancy interruption have recently been developed: (1) the use of prostaglandins for menstrual induction without surgical intervention; and (2) the use of prostaglandins as a cervical priming agent to aid in pregnancy interruption by surgical evacuation. Menstruation has been successfully induced in patients between 5 and 7 weeks of amenorrhea through the use of prostaglandin suppositories alone. Prostaglandins have also been used to soften the cervix prior to suction curettage, or dilatation and evacuation, for surgical termination of more advanced pregnancies. Prostaglandins can aid in averting possible trauma associated with forced mechanical dilatation and instrumentation, and may eventually provide an alternative to surgical interruption at all stages of pregnancy.

MENSTRUAL INDUCTION WITH 15(S)-15-METHYL-PGF$_{2\alpha}$

Historical development

Attempts at using prostaglandins for menstrual induction in early pregnancy began around 1973, when it was found that continuous intravenous administration of prostaglandin $F_{2\alpha}$ ($PGF_{2\alpha}$), at a rate of 50 μg/min for 8 h, aborted the majority of pregnant patients and induced menstrual bleeding in 5 non-pregnant women (Wentz and Jones, 1973). In subsequent studies, serial intramuscular injections of the prostaglandin analog, 15(S)-15-methyl-prostaglandin $F_{2\alpha}$ (15-ME-$PGF_{2\alpha}$), administered at a dose of 250 μg every 2 h for 24 h, successfully terminated pregnancy in 89% of patients with gestations of 5–6 weeks from the last menstrual period (Lauersen and Wilson, 1976).

A major limitation of these techniques, however, was the need for continuous or frequent administration of the prostaglandin. A Silastic device, impregnated with 15-ME-$PGF_{2\alpha}$, developed for vaginal administration, was an early method of providing a measured continuous release of the drug over time. Abortion was successfully induced with this device in 15 of 20 patients in their first trimester, but a 75% success rate, while promising, was not considered clinically acceptable (Lauersen and Wilson, 1977). Further attempts at finding an effective treatment protocol consisted of (1) four 15-ME-$PGF_{2\alpha}$ vaginal suppositories, given at 3 h intervals, which aborted 97% of 75 women in the early first trimester of pregnancy; and (2) a single long-acting wax-based vaginal suppository containing 3 mg of 15-ME-$PGF_{2\alpha}$, which successfully induced abortion in 34 of 39 patients with gestations of 8–19 weeks (Ballard *et al.*, 1978). The use of a single and double 15-ME-$PGF_{2\alpha}$ suppository for menstrual induction was recently investigated by a research team at our institution in a preliminary study of 60 patients, and was found to be effective.

Menstrual induction technique

To terminate early pregnancy (6–8 weeks) through menstrual induction, a single- or double-suppository protocol may be used. In the former technique a single vaginal suppository containing 3 mg of 15-ME-$PGF_{2\alpha}$ in a soluble wax base is inserted in the region of the posterior fornix. With the two-suppository regimen, however, a rapidly acting 1 mg prostaglandin suppository is inserted and followed, after 1–3 h, by the slow-acting 3 mg suppository. Patients are observed in the hospital for 4–10 h before discharge. Although patients are not routinely premedicated with antiemetic and antidiarrheal drugs, these agents can be administered according to the patient's symptoms.

Effects of $PGF_{2\alpha}$ vaginal suppositories

Vaginal administration of 15-ME-$PGF_{2\alpha}$ suppositories can successfully interrupt early pregnancy (Lauersen *et al.*, 1979) with the two-suppository regimen apparently being more effective (95%) than the single-suppository treatment (75%). In the two-suppository group, uterine activity begins at approximately 2 h, $1\frac{1}{2}$ h earlier than the patients receiving a single suppository, although the degree of activity is similar. Vaginal bleeding also starts $1\frac{1}{2}$ h earlier with the two-suppository group, but again, the estimated amount of bleeding is not significantly different (Table 8.1).

Table 8.1 Effects of vaginal prostaglandin

	One suppository	Two suppositories
Uterine activity started	211 ± 93 min	87 ± 61 min
Degree		
Moderate to severe	15	33
None to mild	5	6
Vaginal bleeding started	339 ± 155 min	243.6 ± 133 min
Estimated amount	67 ± 42 ml	58 ± 41 ml
No side-effects	30%	60%
Vomiting	40%	30%
More than one episode	15%	18%
Diarrhea	55%	43%
More than two episodes	15%	18%

Blood level determinations

For research purposes, blood specimens were obtained prior to, and 4, 8 and 10 h subsequent to, the initial prostaglandin administration, and at the time of follow-up. Plasma was tested for levels of 15-ME-PGF$_{2\alpha}$ and serum for HCG and progesterone. Administration of the single long-acting 3 mg suppository resulted in highly variable blood levels of 15-ME-PGF$_{2\alpha}$ at 4, 8 and 10 h. The levels of the prostaglandin detected in the blood frequently dropped after the start of vaginal bleeding. In one patient, vaginal bleeding began within 35 min of the prostaglandin administration, and there were no detectable levels of the analog at 4, 8 and 10 h. This patient had a positive pregnancy test at follow-up (Fig. 8.1A).

The rapidly acting 1 mg suppository followed in 3 h by the longer-acting 3 mg suppository resulted in a more consistent elevation of prostaglandin levels (Fig. 8.1B), and may account for the higher success rate. Neither the single- nor the two-suppository dose schedule produced a consistent or significant decrease in HCG levels during the 10-h observation period. There was a significant drop in progesterone at 4 h with the two-suppository group; however, this drop was transient with recovery by 10 h. There was a decrease in both HCG and progesterone at the time of follow-up in all patients (Fig. 8.2). The seven 'failed' patients, and 14 of the remaining 53 patients, had serum HCG levels at follow-up that might be considered within the pregnant range.

Side-effects of PGF$_{2\alpha}$ suppositories

Patients experience less frequent and less severe gastrointestinal side-effects with the two-suppository regimen, and a number of patients are found to be completely free from side-effects with this regimen ($p < 0.05$) (Table 8.1). Several patients report strong uterine cramping and the passage of clots 2–3 days post-administration but, in general, side-effects are minimal and are well tolerated by patients.

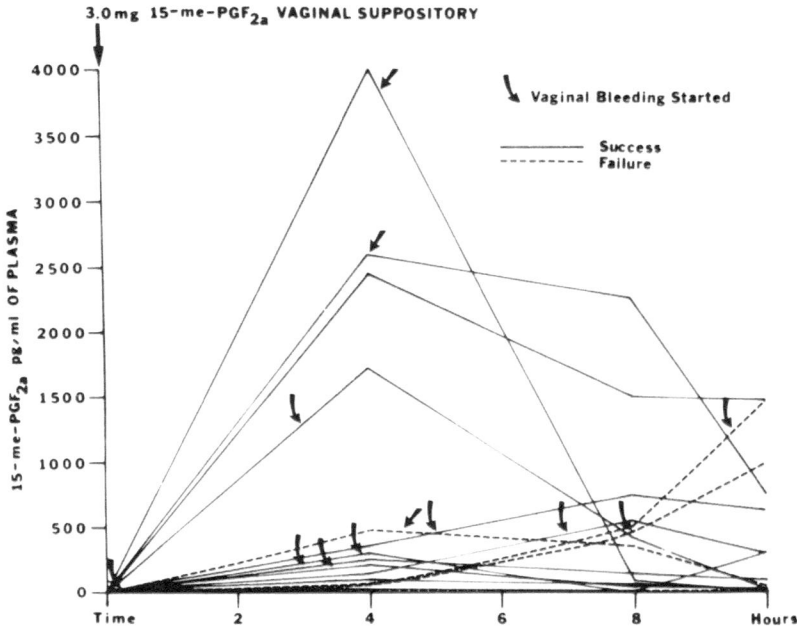

Figure 8.1A Plasma levels of 15-ME-PGF$_{2\alpha}$ as detected by radioimmunoassay following insertion of a 3 mg vaginal suppository

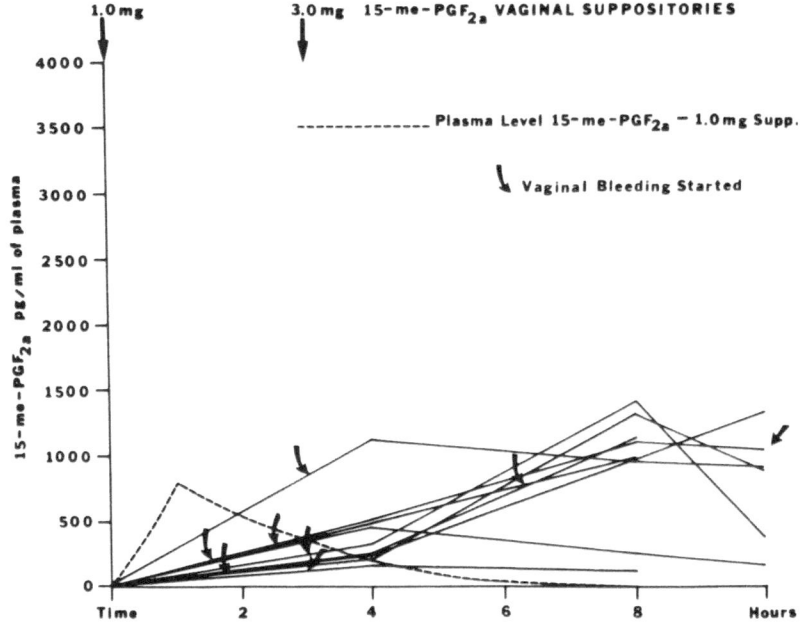

Figure 8.1B Plasma levels of 15-ME-PGF$_{2\alpha}$ as detected by radioimmunoassay following insertion of a 1 mg suppository followed in 3 h by a 3 mg suppository

THE EFFECT OF A 3mg 15-me-PGF₂ₐ VAGINAL SUPPOSITORY IN THE EARLY FIRST TRIMESTER

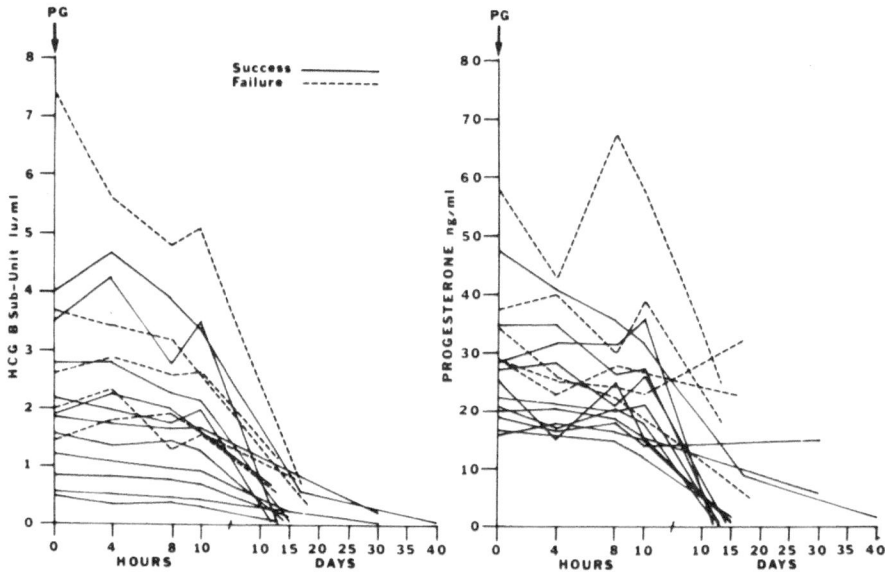

THE EFFECT OF 1mg AND 3mg 15-me-PGF₂ₐ VAGINAL SUPPOSITORIES IN EARLY FIRST TRIMESTER

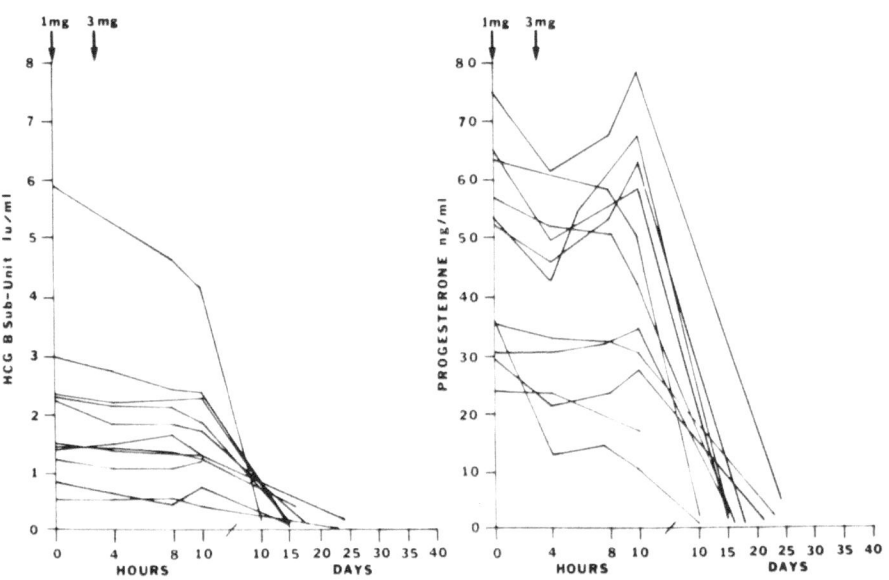

Figure 8.2 Hormonal changes induced by prostaglandin administration. Upper chart represents single suppository group, while lower chart shows effect of a two-suppository regimen

95

PGF$_{2\alpha}$-theoretical mechanism of action

The two-suppository regimen, a rapidly acting 1 mg suppository followed by a long-acting 3 mg suppository, is most effective in the termination of early pregnancy. This double-prostaglandin administration may result in a 'prostaglandin impact' (Caspo et al., 1976) causing the products of conception to be either completely or partially expelled. The long-acting 3 mg suppository alone also successfully terminated pregnancy in 75% of patients (Csapo and Pulkkinen, 1979). However, the two suppositories together appear to have a synergistic effect (Lauersen et al., 1980; Scher et al., 1980).

The initial, transient drop in progesterone observed during the period immediately after suppository insertion appears to be characteristic of prostaglandin administration in early pregnancy (Wentz and Jones, 1973). The significant drop in progesterone and HCG at follow-up may indicate that pregnancy is irreversibly compromised, and a negative urinary HCG might be obtained if suction aspiration is postponed for a period of time. Prolonged elevated serum HCG levels indicate continued presence of trophoblastic tissue, even in view of a negative pregnancy test. When curettage is performed on patients who successfully abort with the 3 mg suppository, necrotic residual tissue is often found at 4 weeks after administration (Mandelin, 1978).

MENSTRUAL INDUCTION WITH THE PGE$_2$ ANALOG – AN ALTERNATIVE METHOD

Historical development

The safety and efficacy of vaginal suppositories containing 9-deoxo-16,16-dimethyl-9-methylene prostaglandin E$_2$ for inducing post-conceptual menses in early pregnancies has recently been tested. Over the last 10 years naturally occurring E$_2$ has been used by investigators for management of abortion, death in utero, and menstrual regulation. Because of the rapid metabolism and inactivation of the natural E$_2$ form, however, it could be administered only by continuous intravenous infusion or repeated administration by other routes. A search was made to develop analogs which would resist rapid metabolism and still maintain biologic activity.

Numerous reports on 15-methyl analogs of PGE$_2$ showed high efficacy rates but, in many cases, there was a significant incidence of gastrointestinal side-effects (Karim, 1975). The prostaglandin analog, 9-deoxo-16,16-dimethyl-9-methylene PGE$_2$ (free acid), was first studied in Sweden and found to have advantageous characteristics such as ease of vaginal administration and reduced gastrointestinal side-effects in post-conceptional menses induction (Bygdeman et al., 1978, 1979). One-third of the patients treated with 75 mg PGE$_2$, repeated after 6 h, resulted in complete abortion, and there was found to be a low incidence of side-effects. Further investigation of this prostaglandin compound seemed warranted to improve the means of early post-conceptional induction of menses.

Menstrual induction technique with PGE$_2$ suppositories

Each patient is given one 9-deoxo-16,16-dimethyl-9-methylene prostaglandin E$_2$ suppository (supplied by the Upjohn Company, Kalamazoo, Michigan) (30 mg) which is inserted high in the vagina in the region of the posterior fornix. After 2h, a larger 75mg vaginal suppository of the same composition is administered. The patient remains in a supine position for a minimum of 30 min following the insertion of each suppository, after which ambulation is permitted. The patients are observed for a period of 4 h following the insertion of the first suppository and then permitted to go home.

Analgesics can be given as needed for discomfort, and the majority of patients receive some pharmaceutical drugs for this purpose. All patients are scheduled for a follow-up visit 14 days after the procedure to ensure that abortion is complete.

Vaginal administration of a 30 and 75 mg 9-deoxo-16,16-dimethyl-9-methylene prostaglandin E$_2$, like administration of the PGF$_{2\alpha}$ analog, successfully induces post-conceptual menses in most patients, with minimal side-effects.

With PGE$_2$ suppositories, uterine activity begins at a mean of $1\frac{1}{2}$ h following treatment (Table 8.1), and bleeding approximately 3–4 h after insertion, though time until menstruation is highly variable (1–9 h).

Side-effects of PGE$_2$ suppositories

Gastrointestinal side-effects are relatively minor with PGE$_2$ administration, and well-tolerated by most patients (Table 8.2). One-third of the women treated are completely free from side-effects with this regimen. For those who do experience side-effects, vomiting, diarrhea, and cramping, are the most common. Occasionally a patient will experience elevation of temperature, or prolonged bleeding following the procedure. Overall, patients report moderate bleeding over an average of 7–8 days.

Table 8.2 Percentages of side-effects of two vaginal PGE$_2$ analog suppositories (30 mg + 75 mg) ($n = 12$)

No side-effects	33
Vomiting	42
More than one episode	33
Diarrhea	33
More than two episodes	25
Cramping (severe)	42
Elevated temperature (101–104˚ F)	8
Prolonged bleeding	8

MENSTRUAL INDUCTION – SUMMARY

Many patients who have had previous pregnancies surgically interrupted, state a preference for termination by the prostaglandin suppository method, and request it again should a subsequent unwanted pregnancy occur. The prostaglandin procedure appears to be less physically and psychologically traumatic than surgical interruption. In general, the side-effects of prostaglandin administration are well tolerated, and are sometimes so minimal that patients report their families and friends did not realize they were undergoing a prostaglandin-induced abortion.

Initial results with vaginal administration of prostaglandin by the two-suppository regimen appear to be very promising. An expanded study is presently under way to determine the practicality of this technique as an out-patient procedure alone. If results remain consistent, a valid pharmacologic alternative to surgical termination of pregnancy may eventually be clinically available.

CERVICAL PRIMING

Introduction

A popular technique for surgical termination of more advanced pregnancies is dilatation and evacuation (D&E). Mid-trimester D&E is gaining increased clinical acceptance, buttressed by reports which demonstrate a significant reduction in maternal morbidity with this technique (Grimes *et al.*, 1977). A persistent problem, however, with both first trimester suction curettage and mid-trimester D&E, is the need for a moderate degree of forceful cervical dilatation to facilitate the removal of the products of conception. Forced cervical dilatation can result in cervical damage and subsequent problems such as spontaneous abortion, incompetent cervical os and premature delivery.

One attempt to minimize the potential for cervical injury present with forceful cervical dilatation has been the use of laminaria tents. These tents, made from dried seaweed, when inserted into the cervical canal, swell to several times the original diameter over a 6–12 h period, dilating the cervix in the process. The technique of laminaria insertion, however, requires skill and is associated with certain problems. The laminaria must be placed well before the planned surgical procedure, for they induce cervical changes by gradually drawing moisture from the surrounding tissue, and this physical phenomenon requires sufficient time. Moreover, side-effects are frequently experienced with the use of laminaria; insertion can be painful, and the patient may experience vaso-vagal symptoms and uterine cramping. Approximately 20% of all patients experience syncope with insertion of laminaria (Eaton *et al.*, 1972) and there is an increased incidence of post-abortion fever and cervical laceration. The laminaria insertion can also injure the cervix by the production of a false tract. Finally, serious problems may develop if the patient does not return to the hospital 24 h after the insertion.

The increasing popularity of surgical interruption of more advanced pregnancies, and the drawbacks in laminaria use, have stimulated a search for improved methods for the production of desired cervical changes prior to surgery. Studies have shown that vaginal administration of prostaglandins, in addition to their ability to induce menstruation and terminate early pregnancies, can also produce cervical dilatation and softening prior to suction curettage. Both the naturally occurring prostaglandins, PGE_2 and $PGF_{2\alpha}$ (Dingfelder et al., 1975), and the 15-methyl analog of $PGF_{2\alpha}$ have been found to be effective in the first trimester for this purpose (Lauersen et al., 1979; Ganguli et al., 1977; Lauersen et al., 1982).

Cervical priming technique

The chosen prostaglandin, either (1) 15(S)-15-methyl-prostaglandin $F_{2\alpha}$ (15-ME-$PGF_{2\alpha}$) (supplied by Glenn D. Gutknecht, The Upjohn Company, Kalamazoo, Michigan) at a dose level of 0.5 mg or 1.0 mg; or (2) 16-dimethyl-9-methylene-prostaglandin E_2 (PGE_2 analog (also supplied by Upjohn Co.) in doses of 30 mg or 60 mg is administered in the form of a vaginal suppository in an 800 mg waxy base. The insertion procedure is simple; the patient is placed in the dorso-lithomic position and a bimanual examination performed to confirm uterine size and determine position. A speculum is then inserted and the cervix steadied with a tenaculum while the degree of pre-existent cervical dilatation is assessed using Hawkins–Ambler dilators. Insertion of the largest dilator should be attempted first, and then the dilator size consecutively reduced until a dilator can be inserted without force. This technique, moving from the larger to the smaller dilator, eliminates any chance of involuntary cervical dilatation during this assessment period. The degree of cervical dilatation can be recorded.

The prostaglandin suppository is digitally inserted high in the vagina in the region of the posterior fornix. The patient should remain in a supine position for 10–15 min after administration, and can then be allowed to ambulate freely. During the entire post-administration period the patient must be carefully observed, and the occurrence of uterine activity, vaginal bleeding or possible side-effects recorded. Prostaglandin suppository administration usually takes place on the day of the scheduled surgery, from 1 to 6 h prior to the surgery. Approximately 10 % of the patients are admitted the night before and receive the prostaglandin at a minimum 12 h before scheduled surgery, though the 30 mg PGE_2 needs to be inserted only 1–2 h before the surgical procedure when gestational age is 9 weeks or less.

If laminaria tents are used, they must be inserted approximately 12 h prior to the dilatation and evacuation procedure. The cervix is packed with four to six laminaria tents and they are removed just prior to the surgical procedure.

Over 9 weeks of gestation, after careful consideration of the stage of the pregnancy and the physical and psychological status of the patient, abortions can be performed under local anesthesia. In these cases the preoperative medication is intravenous diazepam 10 mg and meperidine 100 mg; the local anesthesia is a paracervical block of lidocaine 1 %. Approximately 10 % of patients receive sodium pentothal-induced general anesthesia. The patients under 9 weeks of gestation either do not require premedication or are premedicated with 0.5 cc of 2 % Nubain. At the time of surgery, the degree of cervical dilatation can again be assessed, and if further dilatation is needed it can be achieved with the Hawkins–Ambler dilator. A suction cannula is utilized in all patients for the abortion. In those patients with lower gestational ages, evacuation of the products of conception can frequently be completed with suction alone. More advanced gestations may require a combination of suction and removal of tissue with Bierer and ring forceps. The completeness of the procedure should be checked with sharp curettage in all patients. Oxytocin, 20 units in 500 cc, can be administered intravenously when indicated by the degree of vaginal bleeding. The patient is observed and vital signs checked after the procedure and the patient can usually be discharged within 3–5 h.

Effects of cervical priming with prostaglandin

Vaginal administration of prostaglandin induces some degree of cervical change in all patients; the mean change for late first trimester–early second trimester patients is + 4.2 mm, ranging from + 1 to + 10 mm. However, using 30 mg PGE_2 analog for patients under 9 weeks gestation, the mean change is + 3.1 mm with a range from + 1 to + 7 mm. Administration of the prostaglandins 4–5 h prior to surgery appears to achieve the maximal cervical effect.

The PGE_2 analog is more effective in inducing cervical change than 15-ME-$PGF_{2\alpha}$ for late first trimester–early second trimester pregnancies (Table 8.3). The 30 mg PGE_2 analog appears to be the most clinically useful of the PG suppositories tested, for its administration results in the desired cervical changes with only minimal side-effects. The 60 mg PGE_2 suppository, however, is the most effective on the cervix, but it is felt that the side-effects associated with this dose would limit its clinical acceptability for this indication. In general, the degree of cervical dilatation also appears to increase with the length of the gestation period. Patients with gestations of 14 weeks and higher achieve a mean change in cervical dilatation of approximately 4.4 mm, whereas for those under 9 weeks gestation, mean change in cervical dilatation is around 3.1 mm, significantly lower (Figs 8.3A and 8.3B).

CONCLUDING REMARKS

Vaginal administration of prostaglandin prior to surgical interruption of pregnancy can produce beneficial cervical changes without producing the side-effects associated with the use of laminaria. The cervix not only predilates with prostaglandin, but becomes softer, facilitating further mechanical dilatation when required. The uterus at the time of surgery also appears well contracted, which greatly facilitates the emptying of the uterine contents and minimizes blood loss associated with the procedure. In the more advanced gestations the synergistic effect of prostaglandin and oxytocin is prominent, and aids in the safe evacuation of the uterus.

Though the use of laminaria prior to surgical evacuation may eliminate the need for further dilatation, this technique has been characterized by certain problems to date. Insertion usually must be done on the night before surgery, is

Table 8.3 Results of cervical priming prior to D&E

	15-ME-PGF$_{2\alpha}$		PGE$_2$		PGE$_2$–30 mg (9 weeks gestation or less)
	0.5 mg	1.0 mg	30 mg	60 mg	
No. patients aborted during treatment	0	0	1	1	0
Maternal age (Years ± SDM)	25.1 ± 7.5	22.0 ± 5.6	22.5 ± 7.6	21.4 ± 5.3	22.7 ± 6.3
Cervical changes (mm ± SDM)	3.6 ± 1.9	3.8 ± 1.7	4.4 ± 2.6	4.7 ± 2.7	3.1 ± 1.1
No mechanical dilatation required	25%	20%	30%	40%	88%

often painful, and side-effects are not uncommon. In addition, 25 % of patients with laminaria have a blood loss of more than 200 ml.

The rapid effectiveness of the prostaglandin suppositories (maximal dilatation at approximately 6 h) obviates the need for an overnight hospital stay and eliminates the potential risk that a patient, who perhaps might have had laminaria inserted or a drug administered the night before, would not return for surgery the next morning. The rapid action of the prostaglandin allows cervical priming and the surgical procedure to be performed in the same day; or, at an early gestational stage, prostaglandin can be used to induce menstruation and eliminate the need for surgical intervention entirely.

In examining the side-effects of the various methods, it was found that the overall rate for major complications was higher in the non-prostaglandin abortion patients, (those primed with laminaria or receiving no priming) (Table 8.4). Twenty percent of the non-prostaglandin patients as compared

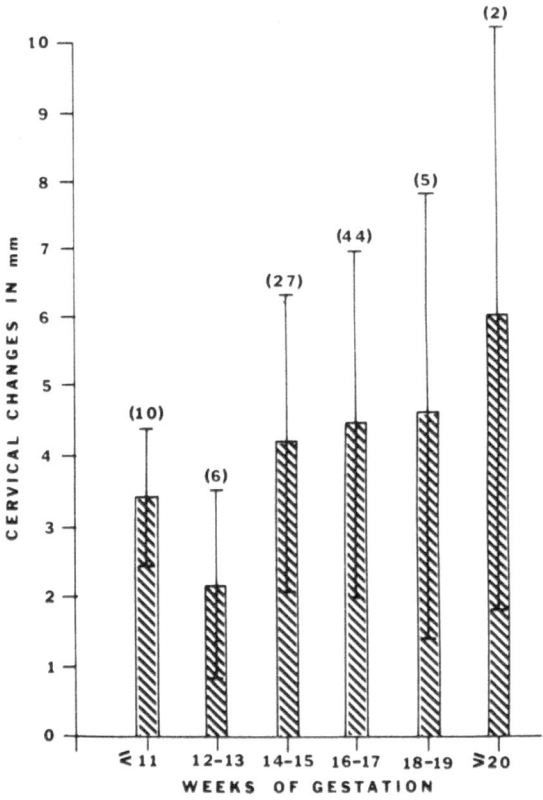

Figure 8.3A The degree of cervical changes induced by preoperative administration of prostaglandin suppositories was plotted against the week of gestation. The results of 95 patients are illustrated by mean and standard deviation of the mean. As gestation increased there was some increase in the amount of induced cervical change, but the prostaglandin appeared to be effective throughout the weeks of gestation tested.

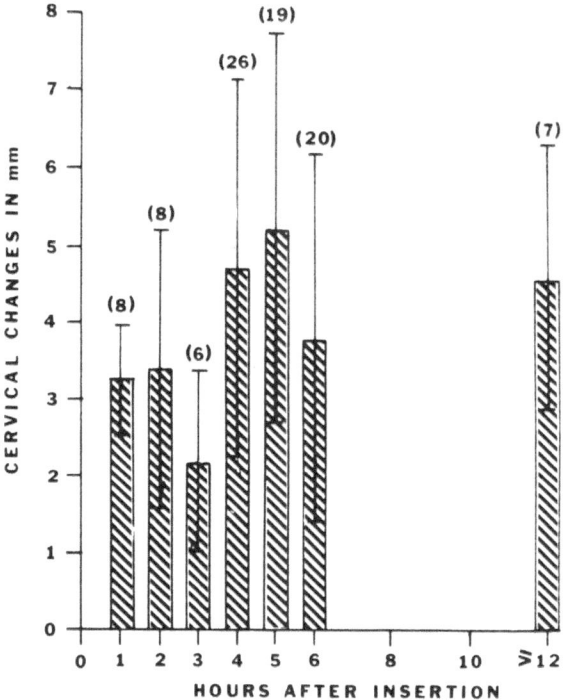

Figure 8.3B The degree of cervical change induced by preoperative administration of prostaglandin suppositories was plotted against the time of administration. The results of 95 patients are illustrated by mean and standard deviation of the mean. Note that the maximal effects appeared at 4 and 5 h, and administration of the suppository more than 12 h prior to surgery did not appear to offer for distinct advantage

with only 1 % of the prostaglandin patients experienced blood loss in excess of 200 ml. Unique to the laminaria patients were the vaso-vagal symptoms of dizziness and fainting on insertion. In addition, 25 % of these patients experienced blood loss in excess of 200 ml, and many developed nausea and vomiting. With prostaglandins, most gastrointestinal side-effects occurred with the higher dosage (60 mg) of the PGE_2 analog, but the majority of the prostaglandin patients were completely free from side-effects.

The use of prostaglandins for menstrual induction in early first trimester, and for softening the cervix prior to surgical intervention in late first trimester—early second trimester pregnancies, represents an innovative approach to improving pregnancy termination techniques. By administering prostaglandins in the manner described in this chapter, pregnancy interruption is facilitated and the need for a costly and inconvenient overnight hospital stay is obviated. Though prostaglandins are still under investigation in this, as in many other areas of application, it appears that their use will continue to increase both as an alternative and an aid to surgical interruption of early

Table 8.4 Side-effects and complications of cervical priming prior to D&E (percentages)

	No priming therapy	Laminaria	15-ME-PGF$_{2\alpha}$		PGE$_2$ analog		PGE$_2$ analog – 30 mg (9 weeks gestation or less)
			0.5 mg	1.0 mg	30 mg	60 mg	
Vomiting	15	10	0	0	8	30	8
Diarrhea	0	0	0	10	3	40	1
Dizziness and fainting	0	15	0	0	0	0	0
Blood loss > 200 ml	15	25	0	0	0	5	0
Cervical laceration	5	0	0	10	0	0	0
Incomplete abortion, second surgery required	5	5	0	0	0	0	1

pregnancy. The proper use of prostaglandins has simplified abortion techniques and greatly increased patient safety. The possibility that the cervical changes induced by the prostaglandin administration will minimize possible harmful, long-term sequelae of the operative procedure, is currently under investigation.

References

Ballard, C. A., Forte, K. and Lauerson, N. H. (1978). Plasma prostaglandin concentration and abortifacient effectiveness of a single insertion of a 3-mg 15(S)-methyl-prostaglandin $F_{2\alpha}$ methyl ester vaginal suppository. *Contraception*, **17**, 383–392

Bygdeman, M., Green, K., Bergstrom, S., Bundy, G. and Kimball, F. A. (1979). A new prostaglandin E_2 analog for pregnancy termination. *Lancet*, **1**, 1136

Bygdeman, M., Martin, J. N., Leader, A., Lundstrom, V., Ramadan, M., Eneroth, P. and Green, K. (1978). Early pregnancy interruption by 15(S) 15 methyl prostaglandin $F_{2\alpha}$ methyl ester. *Obstet. Gynecol.*, **48**, 221–224

Csapo, A. I. and Pulkkinen, M. O. (1979). The mechanism of prostaglandin action on the pregnant human uterus. *Prostaglandins*, **17**, 283–299

Csapo, A. I., Herczeg, J., Pulkkinen, M., Kaihola, H. I., Zoltan, I., Csillag, M. and Mocsary, P. (1976). Termination of pregnancy with double prostaglandin impact. *Am. J. Obstet. Gynecol.*, **135**, 1116

Dingfelder, J. R., Brenner, W. E., Hendricks, C. H. and Staurovsky, L. G. (1975). Reduction of cervical resistance by prostaglandin suppositories prior to dilatation for induced abortion. *Am. J. Obstet. Gynecol.*, **122**, 25–30

Eaton, C. J., Cohn, G. and Bollinger, C. C. (1972). Laminaria tent as a cervical dilator prior to aspiration-type therapeutic abortion. *Obstet. Gynecol.*, **39**, 535–537

Ganguli, A. C., Green, K. and Bygdeman, M. (1977). Preoperative dilatation of the cervix by single vaginal administration of 15-methyl-$PGF_{2\alpha}$-methyl ester. *Prostaglandins*, **14**, 779–784

Grimes, D. A., Schulz, K. F., Cates, W. Jr., and Tyler, C. W. Jr. (1977). Methods of midtrimester abortion: Which is safest? *Int. J. Gynaecol. Obstet.*, **15**, 184–186

Grimes, D. A., Schulz, K. F., Cates, W. Jr. and Tyler, C. W. Jr. (1977). Mid-trimester abortion by dilatation and evacuation – A safe and practical alternative. *N. Engl. J. Med.*, **296**, 1141–1145

Karim, S. M. (ed.) (1975). In: *Prostaglandins and Reproduction*. pp. 77–148

Lauersen, N. H. (1979). Investigation of prostaglandins for abortion. *Acta. Obstet. Gynecol. Scand.*, pp. 1–36

Lauersen, N. H. and Wilson, K. H. (1976). Luteolytic and abortifacient effects of serial intramuscular injections of 15(S)-15-methyl-prostaglandin $F_{2\alpha}$ in early pregnancy. *Am. J. Obstet. Gynecol.*, **124**, 425–429

Lauersen, N. H. and Wilson, K. H. (1977). The effect of a 10-cm², 0.5% 15-ME-$PGF_{2\alpha}$ methyl ester intravaginal silastic device on abortion and plasma prostaglandin concentration. *Prostaglandins*, **13**, 755–762

Lauersen, N. H. and Wilson, K. H. (1980). Early pregnancy interruption with two 15-ME-$PGF_{2\alpha}$ suppositories. *Contraception*, **21**, 273–282

Lauersen, N. H., Kurkulos, M., Graves, Z. R. and Leeds, L. (1982). A new IUD insertion technique utilizing cervical priming with prostaglandin. *Contraception*, **26**, 59–63

Lauersen, N. H., Seidman, S. and Wilson, K. H. (1979). Cervical priming prior to first-trimester suction abortion with a single 15-methyl-prostaglandin-$F_{2\alpha}$ vaginal suppository. *Am. J. Obstet. Gynecol.*, **135**, 1116–1118

Mandelin, M. (1978). Termination of early pregnancy by a single-dose 3.0 mg 15-methyl $PGF_{2\alpha}$ methyl ester vaginal suppository. *Prostaglandins*, **16**, 143–152

Scher, J., Jing, D. Y. and Kerenyi, T. D. (1980). Post-conceptional induction of menses with a single vaginal suppository of 15(S)-15-methyl-prostaglandin $F_{2\alpha}$ methyl ester. *Prostaglandins*, **3**, 469–485

Wentz, A. C. and Jones, G. S. (1973). Intravenous prostaglandin $F_{2\alpha}$ for induction of menses. *Fertil. Steril.*, **24**, 569–577

9
Intra-amniotic prostaglandins for mid-trimester abortion

J. J. AMY

Enzymes controlling the inactivation of natural prostaglandins (PGs) are lacking in amniotic fluid. The half-life time of PGE_2 and $PGF_{2\alpha}$ is therefore considerably longer in the amniotic cavity than in any other body compartment. For $PGF_{2\alpha}$, it would amount to 6–20 h. Amniotic fluid acts as a storage site from which the injected PG is gradually released and it stimulates the myometrium. The means by which this transfer is operated have not been investigated. The amniotic fluid concentration of the oxytocic decreases progressively due – at least intially – to fetal swallowing and inactivation by fetus and placenta. Additional doses of the abortifacient may therefore have to be instilled. Multiple-dose schedules have given higher success rates than single-dose regimens of natural PGs (Karim and Amy, 1975; Karim, 1979).

NATURAL PROSTAGLANDINS

$PGF_{2\alpha}$ has been used either in single (e.g. 50 mg) or in multiple-dose schedules (e.g. 25 mg repeated after 6 h; 40 mg + 20 mg 6 h and 40 mg 24 h after the initial dose). Only few patients were treated with PGE_2 (e.g. 20 mg 24-hourly). In either case, with adequate dosage, 95 % of women aborted within 48 h without additional means being used. The mean time to abortion varied between 14 and 20 h (Karim and Amy, 1975). Data on median induction–abortion intervals and cumulative abortion rates, which are more accurate means of evaluation of the efficacy of abortifacients, are lacking (Edelman et al., 1976).

Due to the slow transfer of PGs across the fetal membranes, and the low levels in maternal plasma, side-effects are less frequent than with other methods of administration. They mainly consist of nausea, vomiting, pyrexia and cramping uterine pain; diarrhea is uncommon. Headache, rigor, chest pain and vasovagal reactions are rare. Bronchospasm and convulsions have occasionally been reported after intra-amniotic injection of $PGF_{2\alpha}$ (Karim and Amy, 1978).

PROSTAGLANDIN ANALOGS

Data concerning the intra-amniotic instillation of PG analogs are summarized in Table 9.1. The 15-methyl analogs and sulprostone have been very efficacious. In more than 90 % of cases a single dose of the drug was sufficient to terminate pregnancy.

COMBINED METHODS

The intravenous infusion of oxytocin, the intracervical insertion of laminaria tents and the intra-amniotic instillation of a hypertonic solution all facilitate PG abortion. But combined methods have serious drawbacks, which explains why their use has not gained more favor (Table 9.2).

Combination of PGF$_{2\alpha}$ and urea

Doses of 5–20 mg PGF$_{2\alpha}$ and 40–80 g urea were simultaneously instilled into the amniotic cavity (Amy, 1979). Due to the use of additional means (e.g. oxytocin and/or laminaria tents) in some of the series, the optimal dose for PGF$_{2\alpha}$ and urea cannot be singled out. With all regimens applied, the induction–abortion interval was markedly shorter (mean of 9–16 h) than that characterizing the sole use of PGF$_{2\alpha}$ intra-amniotically. But gastrointestinal side-effects (up to 70 % of women vomited) and cervical damage requiring repair (up to 3.5 %) occurred more frequently. This could have been caused by a faster systemic absorption of PGF$_{2\alpha}$ from the amniotic cavity, under the influence of urea (Craft et al., 1974; Burkman et al., 1976; Sher and Katz, 1978; Wilson, 1978).

Combination of PGE$_2$ and urea

A shortening of the mean time of abortion, but also a greater frequency of gastrointestinal side-effects and cervical or isthmic damage, are noted when urea is used in conjuction with PGE$_2$. When compared to the intra-amniotic injection of 10 mg PGE$_2$ alone, the combination of 80 g urea and 10 mg PGE$_2$ reduces the mean time to abortion from 27 to 11 h, but vomiting and diarrhea are markedly increased (Craft, 1973). Reducing the dose of PGE$_2$ to 5 or 2.5 mg does not lower the efficacy of the method (95–100 % patients aborted in a mean time of 11 h), but it does not completely abolish the increase in frequency of gastrointestinal intolerance and cervical or isthmic trauma (Bowen-Simpkins, 1973; Craft, 1975).

Combination of PGF$_{2\alpha}$ and hypertonic saline

The combination of 25 mg PGF$_{2\alpha}$ with 200 ml 20 % saline is more efficacious (96 % of subjects aborted within 48 h, in a mean time of 20 h) than either agent

Table 9.1 Termination of pregnancy by intra-amniotic administration of prostaglandin analogs

Compound	Dose	Efficacy	Mean time to abortion (h)	Side-effects (percentage of patients affected or mean number of episodes per patient)	References
15(S),15-methyl-PGE$_2$ methyl ester	100 µg repeated after 24 h	90% in 24 h 100% in 48 h	16.5	Pyrexia (15%) Vomiting (15%)	Amy et al., 1973
15(S),15-methyl-PGF$_{2\alpha}$	2.5 mg single dose	95% in 48 h	18–20	Vomiting (1.3–2.4 episodes) Diarrhea (1.2–1.8 episodes)	Karim and Sivasamboo, 1975; W.H.O. Prostaglandin Task Force, 1976; Krishna et al., 1978; Tejuja et al., 1978
	1.0 mg single dose	92% in 48 h	20.5	Vomiting (0.6 episode) Diarrhea (0.4 episode)	Karim and Sivasamboo, 1975
16,16-dimethyl-PGE$_2$ methyl ester	800 µg single dose	Inadequate stimulation	—	—	Karim and Amy, 1973
Sulprostone	1–4 mg single dose	90–96% in 48 h	17	Vomiting (10%) Diarrhea (5%)	Lichtenegger, 1977; van den Bergh and Haspels, 1978; van den Bergh and Niermeijer, 1979; Schmidt-Gollwitzer et al., 1979

Table 9.2 Accessory means used in conjunction with intra-amniotic prostaglandins for termination of pregnancy

Agent	Dose	Route of administration	Effect
Urea	40–80 g	Intra-amniotic	Enhanced oxytocic effect; Increased intolerance; Increased risk of cervico-isthmic trauma; Increased risk of coagulopathy
NaCl	5–40 g	Intra-amniotic	Id.
Oxytocin	40–120 mU/min	Intravenous	Enhanced oxytocic effect; Increased risk of water intoxication; Increased risk of cervico-isthmic trauma
Calcium gluconate	1–2.75 g	Intra-amniotic	Possibly enhanced oxytocic effect (insufficient data)
Laminaria tents	one or more	Intracervical	Facilitation of cervical dilatation

used alone ($PGF_{2\alpha}$: 68 %; 37 h; NaCl: 52 %; 46 h). In all patients in this study oxytocin was intravenously infused at the rate of 120 mU/min, starting 24 h after intra-amniotic injection (Bostofte *et al.*, 1975).

After intra-amniotic instillation of 20 mg $PGF_{2\alpha}$ and 150–200 ml 20 % saline, oxytocin (40 mU/min) being started at the onset of painful uterine contractions, 99 % of the women expel the fetus vaginally, in a mean time of 17 h. The main side-effect is vomiting (33 %). Hemorrhage and coagulopathy are noted in 2.4 and 1.2 %, respectively (Kerenyi and Den, 1979).

With a lesser salt load (5–10 g, instead of the usual 40 g) injected concomitantly with 20–40 mg $PGF_{2\alpha}$ and oxytocin (40 mU/min) intravenously infused from an early stage on, the mean time to abortion varied between 16 and 22 h (Borten, 1976; Adachi *et al.*, 1977; Muzsnai and Kerenyi, 1979). No modification in the coagulation profile was noted (Muzsnai and Kerenyi, 1979), yet one patient died of hemolysis or disseminated intravascular coagulation, secondary to septicemia (Adachi *et al.*, 1977).

Combination of a prostaglandin and calcium gluconate

The release of activator calcium ions from the sarcoplasmic reticulum into the cytoplasm of the myometrial cell is thought to be the final common step implicated in every process of spontaneous or induced uterine activation (Amy *et al.*, 1984). To enhance the oxytocic properties of the PG 1–2 g calcium gluconate was instilled together with 40 mg $PGF_{2\alpha}$ into the amniotic cavity of 10 patients. There was no control group. All women aborted within 20 h, in a mean time of 14 h. No complication was reported (Weinstein *et al.*, 1976). It is not clear whether the injection of 3 mg sulprostone combined with 2.75 g calcium gluconate is more effective than that of 3 mg of the analog used alone (Van den Bergh and Haspels, 1978).

COMPLICATIONS

Traumatic lesions of the uterus and the cervix

The posterior uterine wall may rupture at the level of the cervico-isthmic junction, due to excessive myometrial stimulation in the presence of an undilating cervix. The lesion presents as a transverse tear through which fetus and placenta are expelled into the vagina. The tear may extend into the lateral aspects of the isthmic region, leading to partial annular detachment of the cervix. Even when repaired, such lesion may fail to heal. Cervico-isthmic rupture is almost exclusively found in young nulliparae and most frequently when the intra-amniotic injection of PG was combined with the use of accessory means (e.g. intra-amniotic urea or intravenous oxytocin) (Bowen-Simpkins, 1973; Duenhoelter and Gant, 1975).

Rupture of the corpus of the uterus has been described in multiparous patients. In about seven cases out of eight rupture occurred after augmentation of the action of the intra-amniotically injected PG by accessory means (Duenhoelter and Gant, 1975; McCarthy and McQueen, 1980).

A third type of lesion, of less consequence, is the longitudinal tear involving the lateral aspect of an insufficiently dilated and non-compliant cervix during expulsion of the conceptus. This lesion is encountered in $1-4\%$ of patients aborted by intra-amniotic injection of a PG, particularly when combined with other agents (Craft, 1975; Burkman et al., 1976).

Administration of a PG by either the extra-amniotic or a systemic route allows for softening and progressive thinning of the cervix to take place. The intra-amniotically injected PG has much less ripening effect on the cervix. Excessive uterine stimulation, in that case, leads to the development of one of the traumatic lesions described.

Convulsions

In a few women given $PGF_{2\alpha}$ by the intra-amniotic route, the electro-encephalogram (EEG) showed transient modifications. This was occasionally accompanied by epileptiform seizures (Grimes et al., 1977; Amy, 1979). A single case of convulsions occurred after the use of PGE_2 (Brash, 1976). The EEG is altered in one-third of subjects given $PGF_{2\alpha}$ intra-amniotically as compared to one-fourth of those treated with hypertonic saline. There is no correlation between electroencephalographic changes and peripheral plasma levels of $PGF_{2\alpha}$ or its principal metabolite. Probably cortical activity is modified during second trimester abortion induced by pharmacological means, irrespective of the agent being used (Shearman et al., 1975).

Disseminated intravascular coagulation

Intra-amniotic instillation of hypertonic solutions promptly causes fetal demise (Sher and Katz, 1978) and pronounced alterations of the chorion, whereupon thromboplastic material is released into the maternal circulation.

Disseminated intravascular coagulation (DIC) ensues, and occasionally leads to hypofibrinogenemia and severe hemorrhage. In PG-induced abortion, no changes in the coagulation profile occur unless a hypertonic solution is used in combination (Karim and Amy, 1975; MacKenzie *et al.*, 1975).

Retention of products of conception

Products of conception are retained in about 40 % of the cases, which is only slightly more frequent than after use of hypertonic solutions (Bygdeman, 1978). It is not a complication *per se*. Exploration of the uterine cavity with a ring forceps or a wide-bore Karman curette, soon after expulsion of the fetus, can safely be done under light intravenous analgesia, should the latter be deemed necessary. Combined with the administration of an ergot derivative this constitutes the best means of prevention of excessive uterine bleeding. It also permits proper assessment of the uterine isthmus and cervix.

Hemorrhage

Excessive blood loss (500 ml and more) is the most frequent complication of interruption of pregnancy by intra-amniotic instillation of PGs (Duenhoelter and Gant, 1975; Nyberg, 1975; Burkman *et al.*, 1976; Bygdeman, 1978; Cates *et al.*, 1978). Hemorrhage occurs after expulsion of the fetus but before that of the placenta. A possible explanation is that myometrial stimulation abates after rupture of the membranes and escape of the amniotic fluid wherein the oxytocic agent is contained.

Maternal death

Eight deaths were associated with the use of intra-amniotic PGs (Adachi *et al.*, 1977; Cates *et al.*, 1977; Tejuja *et al.*, 1978 – see Table 9.3). In each case, death was due to a pre-existing condition, to improper selection of the method of abortion, or to a faulty technique.

COMPARISON WITH OTHER TECHNIQUES OF MID-TRIMESTER ABORTION

Hypertonic saline

In a multicenter randomized study, $PGF_{2\alpha}$ (25 mg repeated after 6 h) was significantly more effective in terminating pregnancy within 48 h (86 % aborted; mean time of 20 h) than 200 ml of 20 % saline (81 %; 30 h). Incomplete abortion (32–34 %) and cervicovaginal fistula (one in each group) occurred with similar frequencies. However, $PGF_{2\alpha}$ was associated with a higher incidence of blood loss of more than 500 ml (4.5 *vs* 1.5 %), vomiting (54 *vs* 19 %) and diarrhea (15 *vs* 1.5 %) (W.H.O. Prostaglandin Task Force, 1976). Edelman *et al.* (1976) treated 372 women by intra-amniotic instillation

Table 9.3 Deaths associated with abortion by intra-amniotic administration of a prostaglandin

Compound	Pre-existing conditions	Cause of death
$PGF_{2\alpha}$[a]	Chronic alcoholism; pancreatitis; pontine myelolysis	Hematemesis + aspiration
$PGF_{2\alpha}$[a]	Severe congestive heart failure	?? Amniotic fluid embolism
$PGF_{2\alpha}$[a]	Chronic hypertension; severe superimposed pre-eclampsia	Hypertensive crisis + cerebral hemorrhage
$PGF_{2\alpha}$[a]	—	Intravenous narcotic + phenothiazine; respiratory arrest
Intravenous oxytocin + intra-amniotic NaCl + intra-amniotic $PGF_{2\alpha}$	—	Septicemia; DIC; acute tubular necrosis
$PGF_{2\alpha} + NaCl$[b]	—	Septicemia; hemolysis or DIC
$PGF_{2\alpha}$[c]	Grand multiparity	Uterine rupture; shock, death during hysterectomy
15-methyl-$PGF_{2\alpha}$[c]	Grand multiparity	Delayed post-abortal bleeding (day 12) shock; death during hysterectomy

[a] Cates et al., 1977; [b] Adachi et al., 1977; [c] Tejuja et al., 1978.

of either $PGF_{2\alpha}$ (50 mg single dose or 25 mg repeated after 6, 24 and 30 h) or hypertonic saline (Table 9.4). Each method resulted in a satisfactory rate of abortions with acceptable frequencies of complications. The multiple 25 mg dose schedule was the most expeditious, and hypertonic saline the least.

Others consider $PGF_{2\alpha}$ given intra-amniotically as more hazardous than hypertonic saline because of an increased risk of heavy uterine bleeding, blood transfusion and surgical evacuation (Grimes et al., 1977; Cates et al., 1978). But, as mentioned above, proper preventive measures considerably reduce the frequency of these complications. Besides, severe complications may follow the use of hypertonic solutions (Karim and Amy, 1975).

Table 9.4 Comparison between intra-amniotic $PGF_{2\alpha}$ and 20 % saline (Edelman et al., 1976).

Responses	50 mg $PGF_{2\alpha}$	25 mg $PGF_{2\alpha} \times 4$	NaCl
Mean time to abortion	20.5 h	17.5 h	26.5 h
Abortion within 24 h	59 %	73 %	43 %
Abortion within 72 h	94 %	98 %	99 %
Incomplete abortion	62 %	66 %	74 %
Vomiting	29 %	42 %	4 %
Diarrhea	15 %	22 %	7 %
Fever (>38 °C)	3 %	8 %	12 %
Convulsion	1 %	0 %	0 %
Blood loss >500 ml	2 %	2 %	2 %
DIC	0 %	0 %	1 %

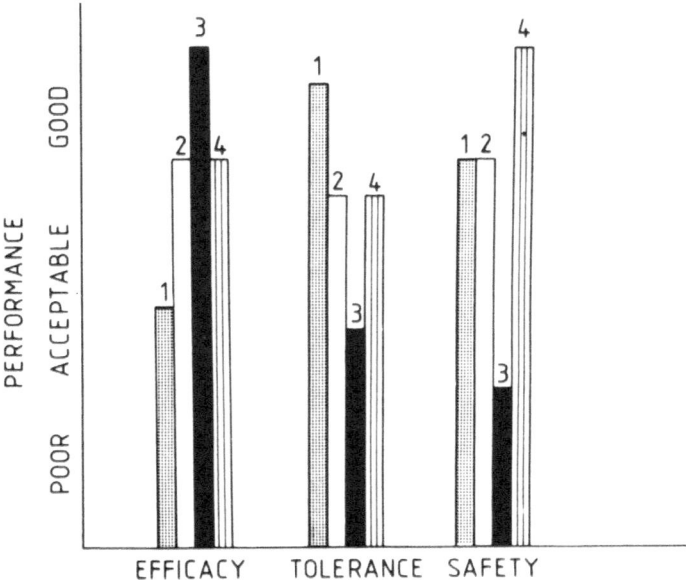

Figure 9.1 Diagrammatic representation of author's views on the efficacy, the tolerance and the safety of various 'pharmacologic' methods of second trimester abortion: (1) intra-amniotic instillation of hypertonic solution; (2) intra-amniotic instillation of prostaglandin; (3) intra-amniotic instillation of hypertonic solution and prostaglandin; (4) systemic administration of one of the recently developed prostaglandin analogs. Overall, the best results are achieved with this latter technique, which also is by far the easiest in its application; but these analogs are not generally available

Dilatation and evacuation

Cadesky *et al.* (1981) consider intracervical insertion of laminaria tents, followed by D&E as safer (7 *vs* 55 % complications) and more expeditious than intra-amniotic instillation of $PGF_{2\alpha}$. However, their study was not randomized and the patients were not matched for gestational length, which was less in the D&E group. Besides, the dosage of $PGF_{2\alpha}$ applied was probably inadequate. Finally, retention of products of conception is not a genuine complication in PG-induced abortion (15 out of 23 'complications' in that group).

Surgical evacuation has not been compared in a randomized fashion with other methods of mid-trimester abortion. Cates *et al.* (1978) and Grimes and Cates (1982) advocate D&E for second trimester termination; but it is associated with a higher incidence of cervical trauma and uterine perforation, and its long-term sequelae in terms of cervical incompetence have yet to be scrutinized.

CONTRAINDICATIONS

Contraindications to transabdominal intrauterine instillation of PGs include:

(1) previous surgery on the uterus;
(2) large uterine fibroids or other pelvic tumors;
(3) major congenital anomalies of the uterus;
(4) grand multiparity;
(5) rupture of the membranes;
(6) fetal death of over 48–72 h duration;
(7) failed saline termination;
(8) hydatidiform mole.

An undue risk of uterine trauma exists in conditions (1) to (4). Yet pregnancy has been successfully terminated by intra-amniotic instillation of a PG in three women with a history of previous cesarean section (Kinra *et al.*, 1977). Rapid absorption of the injected PG with excessive uterine stimulation and severe systemic side-effects, may occur in conditions (6)–(8) (Karim and Amy, 1975).

CONCLUDING REMARKS

The intra-amniotic instillation of a PG requires expertise; it lacks a ripening effect on the cervix and it is associated with a higher incidence of post-abortal hemorrhage. Severe complications occur when cases are improperly selected or when accessory means of uterine stimulation are simultaneously used. Systemic administration of one of the more selective analogs (e.g. sulprostone) presents obvious advantages but these drugs are not available to all (Amy, 1982). We routinely terminate second trimester pregnancy by intra-amniotic instillation of $PGF_{2\alpha}$, according to the following protocol:

(1) Selection of the case.
(2) Ultrasonographic assessment (determination of gestational age; diagnosis of multiple pregnancy or hydatidiform mole; placental localization).
(3) Prophylaxis and treatment of side-effects:
   (a) Loperamide HCl: 4 mg orally prior to the amniocentesis and again 4 h thereafter; 2 mg after each diarrheic stool;
   (b) Haloperidol: 1 mg orally before the amniocentesis and again 8-hourly;
   (c) Meperidine HCl: 100 mg intramuscularly 4-hourly, on demand.
(4) Transabdominal amniocentesis. Slow injection of 50 mg $PGF_{2\alpha}$. Removal of the needle.
(5) Ambulation *ad lib*; liquid diet.
(6) Re-injection of 50 mg $PGF_{2\alpha}$ after 24 h, if needed.
(7) Intravenous infusion of 50 μg/min $PGF_{2\alpha}$, if needed, after spontaneous rupture of the membranes.
(8) Active management of the third stage: expulsion efforts in semi-sitting position + fundal pressure by the assistant; systematic evacuation of

uterine contents + assessment of uterine and cervical integrity within 30 min of fetal expulsion; intramuscular administration of 0.2 mg methyl-ergonovine maleate, unless contraindicated by the existence of hypertension.

(9) D&E in case of failure of expulsion after 48 h.

References

Adachi, A., Wilson, L. and Herzig, N. (1977). Prostaglandin $F_{2\alpha}$ hypertonic saline and oxytocin in midtrimester abortion. *N.Y. State J. Med.*, **77**, 46–49

Amy, J. J. (1979). Interruption de grossesse provoquée par les prostaglandines. In Amy, J. J. (ed.) *Les Prostaglandines et la Reproduction Humaine*. pp. 141–173. (Paris: Flammarion Médecine-Sciences)

Amy, J. J. (1982). Termination of second trimester pregnancy with prostaglandin analogues. In Keirse, M. J. N. C., Bennebroek Gravenhorst, J., van Lith, D. A. F. and Embrey, M. P. (eds). *Second Trimester Pregnancy Termination*. pp. 115–131. (The Hague: Leiden University Press)

Amy, J. J., De Brucker, P. and Merckx, M. (1984). Control of uterine activity in pregnancy. In Hafez, E. S. E. (ed.), *Spontaneous Abortion*. (Lancaster: MTP Press)

Amy, J. J., Karim, S. M. M. and Sivasamboo, R. (1973). Intra-amniotic administration of prostaglandin 15(S), 15-methyl-E_2 methyl ester for termination of pregnancy. *J. Obstet. Gynecol. Br. Commonw.*, **80**, 1017–1020

van den Bergh, A. S. and Haspels, A. A. (1978). Termination of second trimester pregnancy with intra-amniotic administration of 16-phenoxy-ω-tetranor-PGE_2-methyl-sulfonamide (SHB 286) alone and combined with oxytocin and calcium gluconate. *Contraception*, **18**, 635–639

van den Bergh, A. S. and Niermeijer, O. (1979). Termination of advanced second trimester pregnancy with intra-amniotic sulprostone. In Friebel, K., Schneider, A. and Würfel, H. (eds.) *International Sulprostone Symposium*, pp. 119–126. (Berlin: Schering AG)

Borten, M. (1976). Use of combination prostaglandin $F_{2\alpha}$ and hypertonic saline for midtrimester abortion. *Prostaglandins*, **12**, 625–630

Bostofte, E., Stakemann, G. and Stocklund, K. E. (1975). A comparison of termination of pregnancies in the 2nd trimester induced by intra-amniotic injection of hypertonic saline, prostaglandin $F_{2\alpha}$ or both drugs. *Acta Obstet. Gynecol. Scand.*, Suppl. 37, 47–50

Bowen-Simpkins, P. (1973). The induction of second trimester abortion using an intra-amniotic injection of urea and prostaglandin E_2. *J. Obstet. Gynaecol. Br. Commonw.*, **80**, 824–826

Brash, J. H. (1976). A generalized epileptiform convulsion after intra-amniotic prostaglandin E_2. *Br. J. Obstet. Gynaecol.*, **83**, 665–666

Burkman, R. T., Atienza, M. F., King, T. M. and Burnett, L. S. (1976). Intra-amniotic urea and prostaglandin $F_{2\alpha}$ for midtrimester abortion: A modified regimen. *Am. J. Obstet. Gynecol.*, **126**, 328–333

Bygdeman, M. (1978). Comparison of prostaglandin and hypertonic saline for termination of pregnancy. *Obstet. Gynecol.*, **52**, 424–429

Cadesky, K. I., Ravinsky, E. and Lyons, E. R. (1981). Dilation and evacuation: A preferred method of midtrimester abortion. *Am. J. Obstet. Gynecol.*, **139**, 329–332

Cates, W. Jr., Grimes, D. A., Haber, R. J. and Tyler, C. W. Jr. (1977). Abortion deaths associated with the use of prostaglandin $F_{2\alpha}$. *Am. J. Obstet. Gynecol.*, **127**, 219–222

Cates, W. Jr., Grimes, D. A., Schulz, K. F., Ory, H. W. and Tyler, C. W. Jr. (1978). World Health Organization studies of prostaglandins versus saline as abortifacients – a reappraisal. *Obstet. Gynecol.*, **52**, 493–498

Craft, I. (1973). Induction of abortion by combined intra-amniotic urea and prostaglandin E_2 or prostaglandin E_2 alone. *Lancet*, **1**, 1344–1346

Craft, I. (1975). Intra-amniotic urea and low-dose prostaglandin E_2 for mid-trimester termination. *Lancet*, **1**, 1115–1116

Craft, I., Walker, E. and Youssefnejadian, E. (1974). Intra-amniotic prostaglandin $F_{2\alpha}$ and urea for abortion. *Prostaglandins*, **5**, 397–407

Duenhoelter, J. H. and Gant, N. F. (1975). Complications following prostaglandin $F_{2\alpha}$-induced midtrimester abortion. *Obstet. Gynecol.*, **46**, 247–250

Edelman, D. A., Brenner, W. E., Mehta, A. C., Philips, F. S., Bhatt, R. V. and Bhiwandiwala, P. (1976). A comparative study of intra-amniotic saline and two prostaglandin $F_{2\alpha}$ dose schedules for midtrimester abortion. *Am. J. Obstet. Gynecol.*, **125**, 188–195

Grimes, D. A. and Cates, W. Jr. (1982). Instrumental abortion in the second trimester: an overview. In Keirse, M. J. N. C., Bennebroek Gravenhorst, J., van Lith, D. A. F. and Embrey, M. P. (eds.) *Second Trimester Pregnancy.* pp. 65–79. (The Hague: Leiden University Press)

Grimes, D. A., Schulz, K. F., Cates, W. Jr. and Tyler, C. W. Jr. (1977). Midtrimester abortion by intra-amniotic prostaglandin $F_{2\alpha}$ safer than saline? *Obstet. Gynecol.*, **49**, 612–616

Karim, S. M. M. (1979). Termination of second trimester pregnancy with prostaglandins. In Karim, S. M. M. (ed.). *Advances in Prostaglandin Research – Practical Applications of Prostaglandins and their Synthesis Inhibitors*, pp. 375–409. (Lancaster: MTP Press)

Karim, S. M. M. and Amy, J. J. (1973). Effect of prostaglandin 16,16 dimethyl E_2 methyl ester on the pregnant human uterus. *Prostaglandins.* **4**, 581–592

Karim, S. M. M. and Amy, J. J. (1975). Interruption of pregnancy with prostaglandins. In Karim, S. M. M. (ed.). *Advances in Prostaglandin Research – Prostaglandins and Reproduction.* pp. 77–148. (Lancaster: MTP Press)

Karim, S. M. M. and Amy, J. J. (1978). Prostaglandins and human reproduction. In Macdonald, R. R. (ed.). *Scientific Basis of Obstetrics and Gynecology*, 2nd edn. pp. 345–392. (Edinburgh: Churchill Livingstone)

Karim, S. M. M. and Sivasamboo, R. (1975). Termination of second trimester pregnancy with intra-amniotic 15(S)15 methyl prostaglandin $F_{2\alpha}$ – a two dose schedule study. *Prostaglandins*, **9**, 487–494

Kerenyi, T. D. and Den, T. (1979). Intra-amniotic instillation of saline and prostaglandin for midtrimester abortion. In Zatuchni, G. I., Sciarra, J. J. and Speidel, J. J. (eds.), *Pregnancy Termination – Procedures, Safety, and New Developments*, pp. 254–260. (Hagerstown: Harper and Row)

Kinra, G., Argawal, N. and Hingorani, V. (1977). Use of prostaglandin for induction of second trimester abortions in high risk pregnancy. *Contraception*, **16**, 243–255

Krishna, U., Ganguli, A. C., Mandlekar, A. V. and Purandare, V. N. (1978). Administration of prostaglandins by various routes for induction of abortion; merits and demerits. *Prostaglandins*, **15**, 685–693

Lichtenegger, W. (1977). Abortinduktion mit Prostaglandin $F_{2\alpha}$ und einem neuen Prostaglandin-E_2-Derivat. *Wiener Med. Wochenschr.*, **17**, 536–538

MacKenzie, I. Z., Sayers, L. and Bonnar, J. (1975). Coagulation changes during second-trimester abortion induced by intra-amniotic prostaglandin E_2 and hypertonic solutions. *Lancet*, **2**, 1066–1069

McCarthy, T. and McQueen, J. (1980). Uterine rupture as a complication of second trimester abortion using intra-amniotic prostaglandin E_2 and augmentation with other oxytocic agents. *Prostaglandins*, **19**, 849–854

Muzsnai, D. and Kerenyi, T. (1979). Use of prostaglandin, hypertonic saline and oxytocin for second-trimester abortion. *Eur. J. Obstet. Gynecol. Reprod. Biol.*, **9**, 385–389

Nyberg, R. (1975). Intra-amniotic administration of prostaglandin $F_{2\alpha}$ for therapeutic abortion. *Acta Obstet. Gynecol. Scand.*, Suppl. **37**, 41–46

Schmidt-Gollwitzer, M., Schuessler, B., Schmidt-Gollwitzer, K. and Nevinny-Stickel, J. (1979). Recommendations for the treatment of induction of abortion with sulprostone. In Friebel, K., Schneider, A. and Würfel, H. (eds.) *International Sulprostone Symposium.* pp. 112–126. (Berlin: Schering AG)

Shearman, R. P., Lyneham, R. C., Walsh, J. C., Itzkowic, D. and Shutt, D. A. (1975). Electroencephalographic changes after intra-amniotic prostaglandin $F_{2\alpha}$ and hypertonic saline. *Br. J. Obstet. Gynaecol.*, **82**, 314–317

Sher, G. and Katz, M. (1978). Midtrimester intra-amniotic administration of prostaglandin $F_{2\alpha}$ in combination with a hyperosmolar urea solution: effect upon plasma levels of estradiol, progesterone, and human placental lactogen (HPL). *Acta Obstet. Gynecol. Scand.*, **57**, 223–225

Tejuja, S., Choudhury, S. D. and Manchanda, P. K. (1978). Use of intra- and extra-amniotic prostaglandins for the termination of pregnancies. Reports of multicentric trial in India. *Contraception*, **18**, 641–652

Weinstein, L., Droegemueller, W. and Greer, B. (1976). The synergistic effect of calcium and prostaglandin $F_{2\alpha}$ in second trimester abortion. *Obstet. Gynecol.*, **48**, 469–471

W.H.O. Prostaglandin Task Force (1976). Comparison of intra-amniotic prostaglandin $F_{2\alpha}$ and hypertonic saline for induction of second-trimester abortion. *Br. Med. J.*, **1**, 1373–1376

Wilson, W. B. Jr. (1978). Midtrimester abortion with urea, prostaglandin $F_{2\alpha}$, laminaria and oxytocin. A new regimen. *Obstet. Gynecol.*, **51**, 699–701

10
Intramuscular administration of 15-methyl prostaglandin $F_{2\alpha}$ and laminaria insertion for termination of mid-trimester pregnancy

S. D. SHARMA, V. M. STEINMILLER and R. W. HALE

INTRODUCTION

Termination of mid-trimester pregnancy remains a significant clinical problem. In order to avoid operative procedures such as hysterotomy, a number of techniques for the induction of uterine activity resulting in spontaneous expulsion of products of conception are being investigated. Since the 1970s the naturally occurring prostaglandins E_2 and $F_{2\alpha}$ have been used to terminate pregnancy (Karim and Filshie, 1970; Bygdeman and Wiqvist, 1971; Embrey, 1971). Naturally occurring prostaglandins E_2 and $F_{2\alpha}$ are rapidly metabolized and inactivated in the body. They must be given by continuous intravenous infusion or by repeated administration via other routes such as intrauterine, vaginal or intramuscular methods. The introduction of the methyl group in the 15 position of the prostaglandins E_2 and $F_{2\alpha}$ protects them against enzymatic degradation by prostaglandin 15-dehydrogenase, thus prolonging their duration of action and their potency (Bundy *et al.*, 1971; Yankee and Bundy, 1972). The clinical application of these analogs to terminate pregnancy was first reported by Karim and Sharma (1972). The analog 15(S)-15-methyl-prostaglandin $F_{2\alpha}$ (15-me-$PGF_{2\alpha}$), unlike the naturally occurring $PGF_{2\alpha}$ can be given intramuscularly without causing local inflammation or severe pain at the site. It also has a practical advantage in patients with ruptured membranes in mid-trimester pregnancy. 15-me-$PGF_{2\alpha}$ has an overall potency of approximately ten to twenty times that of $PGF_{2\alpha}$. A large number of clinical trials have been carried out since 1972 to evaluate the usefulness of intramuscular 15-me-$PGF_{2\alpha}$ for termination of mid-trimester pregnancy (WHO Multicenter Study, 1977). While the efficacy of 15-me-$PGF_{2\alpha}$ is not in doubt, the incidence of gastrointestinal side-effects, such as nausea, vomiting, and diarrhea, are too high and in unacceptable ranges. In order to reduce the severity of gastrointestinal side-effects, antidiarrheals and antiemetics are recommended routinely as premedication and during the procedure. The side-effects can also be minimized by shortening the injection–abortion interval by the use of laminaria tents 12–18 h prior to the administration of 15-me-PGF$_{2\alpha}$ (Sharma *et al.*, 1975; Stubblefield *et al.*, 1976). The use of laminaria has also reduced the number of serious cervical lacerations (Duenhoelter *et al.*, 1976; Stubblefield *et al.*, 1975).

The following is an evaluation of our experience with intramuscular 15-me-PGF$_{2\alpha}$ combined with laminaria insertion for termination of mid-trimester pregnancy at Kapiolani/Children's Medical Center.

MATERIALS AND METHODS

Patient selection

Intramuscular 15-me-PGF$_{2\alpha}$ was given to 605 women between 1976 and 1982 at Kapiolani/Children's Medical Center. From 1976 to 1978 it was given under close supervision by one investigator as a research study. In January 1979, 15-me-PGF$_{2\alpha}$ was approved by the United States of America's Food and Drug Administration, becoming available to all practicing gynecologists. Although the patients were supervised by different gynecologists throughout this period, the same protocol was utilized. The mean age of these patients was 23.4 years (range 13–43), the mean weight, 55.1 kg. Of these, 490 were admitted desiring termination of pregnancy, 67 with ruptured membranes and 48 women with intrauterine fetal demise. Gestational age was calculated from the first day of last menstrual period. Parity and gestational age of these patients are shown in Table 10.1.

Prior to the procedure a full history was taken and a complete examination, including a pelvic examination, was performed. Written informed consent was obtained from all the patients or their guardians.

Table 10.1 Parity and gestational age of patients treated with 15 me-PGF$_{2\alpha}$

	Termination of pregnancy	Ruptured membrane	IUFD*
Parity			
Nulliparous	276	36	10
Para 1–4	183	30	32
Para 5 and above	31	1	6
Total	490	67	48
Gestational age in weeks			
14–16	112	4	6
17–20	358	42	22
21–24	20	21	20
Total	490	67	48

* Intrauterine fetal demise

Laboratory tests

The minimum laboratory workup included the following: complete blood count, blood group and typing for Rh (D) antigen and urinalysis. In patients with intrauterine fetal demise, blood coagulation studies were performed.

Laminaria insertion

The day prior to prostaglandin administration, one to four laminarias were inserted into the cervical canal of each patient. In 17 patients the cervix was tightly closed and only one small laminaria could be initially inserted. In these cases the laminaria was removed after 6–8 h and replaced by larger, or more than one, laminarias. The laminarias were inserted either in the outpatient clinic or in the hospital, and left in place for 2–36 h, with a mean duration of 18 h. The pelvic examination was carried out on all of the patients immediately prior to the administration of 15-me-PGF$_{2\alpha}$, at which time the laminarias were removed and cervical dilatation evaluated.

Premedication

At approximately 1–2 h prior to the administration of 15-me-PGF$_{2\alpha}$ injection, premedication included dephenoxylate hydrochloride 5 mg with atropine sulfate 0.05 mg orally and prochlorperazine 10 mg intramuscularly. These were repeated every 2–6 h as required.

Dosage schedule of 15-me-PGF$_{2\alpha}$

250 μg of me-PGF$_{2\alpha}$ was administered deep into the gluteal muscle and repeated every 2 h until the fetus and placenta were expelled. In 19 patients the drug was discontinued during the night to allow the patients to sleep, and restarted in the morning.

Uterine curettage

Pelvic examination in lithotomy position was carried out within 2 h after the expulsion of fetus and placenta or the fetus only. At this time, if the placenta was lying in the vagina or in the cervical canal, it was removed manually or with sponge forceps. Uterine curettage was performed routinely in all cases without general anesthesia. In instances when it was not possible to remove the placenta with sponge forceps, 15-me-PGF$_{2\alpha}$ was continued for another 4–6 h. During this period, if the placenta failed to separate, uterine evacuation was carried out under general anesthesia.

Observation during the procedure

Vital signs – heart rate, respiration, temperature and blood pressure – were carefully monitored and recorded. The occurrence of uterine cramps, vaginal bleeding and side-effects were noted. Vaginal examination was carried out when necessary. Estimated blood loss during the procedure was recorded.

Interpretation of results

Success was considered when the products of conception were expelled in their entirety or could be removed manually or with sponge forceps. Incomplete abortion was defined as partial expulsion of the products of conception from the uterus, necessitating surgical evacuation.

Injection to abortion time (IAT) was defined as the interval from the first injection of intramuscular 15-me-PGF$_{2\alpha}$ to the expulsion of the fetus and placenta.

RESULTS

Of the 490 patients for termination of pregnancy, 366 (75 %) aborted within 12 h and 484 (98.7 %) within 48 h (Table 10.2). The mean IAT was 12.6 h. The age, weight and parity of these patients did not influence the IAT in this study. The duration of time the laminaria was in place ranged between 2 and 36 h, with a mean of 17.8 h. In 14 cases, at the time of laminaria removal, it was noted that the laminaria failed to traverse the internal cervical os. In these cases, the IAT was over 18 h. Six patients failed to abort after 48 h, 15-me-PGF$_{2\alpha}$ was continued in four of these patients with successful outcomes. In two cases the cervix was sufficiently dilated so that surgical evacuation of products of conception was carried out without any problems.

The placenta was expelled spontaneously in 211 (43 %) of patients and was removed manually or with the sponge forceps in 269 (55 %) of the cases. Ten patients required general anesthesia for placental removal and placenta accreta was diagnosed in two cases. In the majority of women, only decidual tissue was removed on routine curettage.

Table 10.2   Injection—abortion interval (IAT) with intramuscular 15-me-PGF$_{2\alpha}$

IAT	Termination of pregnancy (mid-trimester)		Patients with ruptured membranes		Intrauterine fetal demises	
	No. of cases	Percentage	No. of cases	Percentage	No. of cases	Percentage
0–6 h	95	19	39	58	30	62.5
7–12 h	271	55	20	30	10	21
13–24 h	110	23	6	9	5	10.5
25–48 h	8	2	2	3	3	6
49 h or more	6	1	—	—	—	—
Total	490	100	67	100	48	100

Cases with ruptured membranes

41 patients in this group initially had intra-amniotic instillation of PGF$_{2\alpha}$ for termination of pregnancy. In these patients premature rupture of membranes occurred with the loss of intra-amniotic drug and lack of, or insufficient, uterine activity. All of these patients had laminaria insertion prior to instillation of intra-amniotic prostaglandin. Twenty-six patients had spontaneous rupture of membranes between 16 and 24 weeks gestation. None of these patients had laminaria insertion. In this group, the IAT varied between 2 and 44 h; 39 patients (58 %) aborted within 6 h and 20 (30 %) within 12 h (Table 10.2). None of these patients required placental removal under general anesthesia.

Intrauterine fetal demise

All 48 patients with intrauterine fetal demise aborted within 48 h. The cumulative abortion rates at 12 and 24 h were 83.5 % and 94 % respectively. The products of conception were expelled completely with amniotic sac intact in 39 cases. The remaining nine required manual removal of the placenta from the vagina or cervical canal. All of these patients had laminaria insertion. None of the patients had coagulation disorders.

Estimated blood loss during and after expulsion of the products of conception was between 60 and 300 ml. Only three patients had blood loss of more than 500 ml, and none required blood transfusion.

Most of the patients experienced lower abdominal pain or discomfort due to uterine contractions within 30 min of intramuscular 15-me-PGF$_{2\alpha}$ administration. Each patient was individualized for analgesic needs.

It is important to evaluate these patients by vaginal examinations frequently. In a number of cases, without the patient's awareness, the fetus, with or without the placenta, was found lying in the vagina. This is more likely to happen during the night. The main side-effects (Table 10.3) with intramuscular 15-me-PGF$_{2\alpha}$ were nausea, vomiting, and diarrhea. These symptoms were somewhat alleviated with liberal use of antiemetic and antidiarrheal drugs. At no time was it necessary to terminate 15-me-PGF$_{2\alpha}$ therapy because of the side-effects. Fifty-four women had temperature elevations of more than 2°F above pre-treatment level. Only 21 of these required antibiotic treatment. In the remainder, the temperature returned to normal within 6 h after the last dose of 15-me-PGF$_{2\alpha}$. None of the other side-effects (Table 10.3) required special treatment. Three patients had minor cervical lacerations which did not require suturing.

There were 11 patients with histories of one previous cesarean section, and four patients with histories of two cesarean sections. In these 15 cases pregnancy was successfully terminated.

Sixty-one patients stayed in the hospital for less than 24 h and 41 for more than 48 h. In the remaining 496 cases, the length of the stay in the hospital was between 24 and 48 h.

Fourteen patients were readmitted to the hospital 2–10 days after the procedure; five required uterine curettage for incomplete abortion and nine

Table 10.3 Side-effects and complications with intramuscular 15-me-PGF$_{2\alpha}$

Side-effects	Patients	
	No.	Percentage
Emesis	369	61
No. of episodes (2–11)		
Mean 1.8		
Diarrhea	417	69
No. of episodes (1–11)		
Mean 2.4		
Temp. elevation >100.4°F	54	9
Infection	21	3.5
Chills and shivering	22	4
Flushing of skin	21	3
Chest pain or tightness	12	2
Shortness of breath	25	4
Dyspnea	30	5
Headache	19	3
Bradycardia	32	5
(less than 20/min from initial rate)		
Tachycardia	24	4
(more than 20/min from initial rate)		
Blood loss more than 500 ml	3	Less than one
Cervical lacerations	3	Less than one

were treated for pelvic infection. This procedure was well tolerated and accepted by the patients.

DISCUSSION

The analog 15-me-PGF$_{2\alpha}$ given intramuscularly for termination of mid-trimester pregnancy has been extensively studied since its use was first reported (Karim and Sharma, 1972). In our study, 98.7% of the patients aborted within 48 h. These results compare favorably with other investigators (Table 10.4). Success rates between 85% and 100% have been reported by various investigators (Table 10.4). Only six patients failed to abort within 48 h; four of these were successfully completed by continuing administration of intramuscular 15-me-PGF$_{2\alpha}$. The remaining two had surgical evacuation carried out under general anesthesia without problems.

The placenta was spontaneously expelled by 43% of the women and was removed manually or with sponge forceps in the other 55%. We agree with Berger and Kerenyi (1974 a,b), that spontaneous expulsion of the placenta mostly occurs within 2 h of the abortion of the fetus. Patients should be routinely examined within 2 h of abortion for placental removal, if not already delivered, as well as inspection of the cervix for lacerations. Only three patients had blood loss of more than 500 ml. The bleeding in these cases occurred after the delivery of the fetus and prior to the placental expulsion. This bleeding may have been due to partial separation of the placenta. None of the patients required blood transfusion. 15-me-PGF$_{2\alpha}$ was found to be a

Table 10.4 Termination of pregnancy with intramuscular 15-me-PGF$_{2\alpha}$

Reference	No. of women	Dosage	IAT	Percentage effective
Bygdeman et al. (1974)	30	250–500 µg 3 hourly	16.1	100
Lauersen and Wilson (1975)	35	250 µg/2 h for 24 h	16	100
World Health Organization (1977)	512	250 µg then 300 µg/3 h	N/P 15.7/13.7	85
Lange and Secher (1977)	80	250 µg/12 h	N/P 18.2/16.4	98
Schwallie et al. (1979)	815	Variable 100–500 µg/1–3 h interval 250–500 µg/ 1½–3½ h interval	15.8	85–94
Sharma et al. (present study)	490	250 µg/2 h	12.6	98.7*

N = Nulliparous; P = parous
* All patients had laminaria insertion

very effective uterotonic agent. Most of the patients did not require an oxytocic agent after the procedure.

In 1975, the study with intramuscular 15-me-PGF$_{2\alpha}$ with and without laminaria insertion (Sharma et al., 1975) was reported. The IAT was longer in patients without laminaria compared to women with laminaria insertion. Similar results have been reported by other investigators (Brenner et al., 1973; Stubblefield et al., 1974; Berman et al., 1974; Globus et al., 1976). Laminaria insertion facilitates mid-trimester termination of pregnancy by shortening the IAT, thereby reducing the complications and side-effects associated with intramuscular 15-me-PGF$_{2\alpha}$. Further, it reduces the incidence of serious cervical lacerations (Stubblefield et al., 1975; Duenhoelter et al., 1976). In this study, only three patients had minor cervical lacerations and none required suturing. One of the concerns with laminaria insertion is whether this procedure increases the risk of infection. Several investigators have reported a lower incidence of infection when laminarias were combined with PGF$_{2\alpha}$ (Duenhoelter et al., 1976; Stubblefield et al., 1974, 1975), whereas a higher incidence of endometritis has been reported by other investigators (Gruber, et al., 1976; Lischke, and Goodling 1973). In this study only 21 patients (3.5 %) were treated for infection and later nine were readmitted for treatment of pelvic infection. For laminaria to be effective, proper placement is essential. When the laminaria did not traverse the cervical internal os, cervical dilatation was ineffective. The laminarias failed to traverse the internal os in 14 women. Subsequently, these patients had prolonged IAT. In similar cases it might be beneficial to replace the laminaria and postpone the procedure for 12 h.

We feel that the patient's length of stay in the hospital could be shortened by inserting laminarias in the physician's office or the outpatient department the day prior to her admission to the hospital for the procedure.

Intramuscular 15-me-PGF$_{2\alpha}$ was found to be very effective in two groups of women, one group with spontaneous rupture of membranes, and the other having had intra-amniotic instillation of $PGF_{2\alpha}$ initially and during the course of the procedure had ruptured membranes. All of these women aborted within 48 h, the IAT was shorter in both of these groups (Table 10.2). Success rates between 90 % and 100 % have been reported (Corson and Bolognese, 1979; Laursen and Wilson, 1977; Schwallie et al., 1980) in women who failed to abort with other methods. It is felt that in these types of cases, intramuscular 15-me-$PGF_{2\alpha}$ is very useful to complete the abortion. It is an effective alternative to oxytocin infusion or surgery.

The recognition of coagulation disorders in patients with intrauterine fetal demise has led to active management in these cases. Intravenous oxytocin is often unsuccessful. In addition, the high dosage of oxytocin required may result in water intoxication and convulsions (Liggins, 1962). Prostaglandin given by various routes has proven very effective in the management of intrauterine fetal demise. The intra-amniotic instillation of prostaglandin subjects the patient to the potential hazards of the technique of amniocentesis and also to the risk of infection. The vaginal route of prostaglandin administration has also been successfully employed (Southern et al., 1978). A disadvantage of the vaginal route is that the absorption of the drug may be interfered with in patients with vaginal bleeding or ruptured membranes. Intramuscular 15-me-$PGF_{2\alpha}$ combined with laminaria insertion offers a safe and reliable means of terminating pregnancy after intrauterine fetal demise.

The efficacy of intramuscular 15-me-$PGF_{2\alpha}$ as an abortifacient is not in doubt, but the very high incidence of gastrointestinal side-effects is unacceptable both to the physicians and the patients. These side-effects are due to the rapid rise in plasma levels of 15-me-$PGF_{2\alpha}$, 15–20 min after its administration (Green and Bygdeman, 1977). Premedication with an antiemetic and an antidiarrheal, followed by routine use during the procedure, decreases the incidence and frequency of these symptoms (Sharma et al., 1975). In this series, 61 % and 69 % of patients experienced vomiting and diarrhea respectively (Table 10.3). The number of episodes of vomiting and diarrhea was markedly reduced with mean of 1.8 (vomiting) and 2.4 (diarrhea) in this series. Thus, by reducing the frequency of these symptoms, the procedure was well accepted by the patients. Other side-effects (Table 10.3) did not require special treatment. The laboratory tests did not show any significant changes.

The abortion was successfully accomplished in 15 cases with previous cesarean section. These patients require frequent evaluation during and after the procedure for evidence of rupture-uterus.

At no time did the side-effects necessitate the termination of therapy. Intramuscular injection caused very little discomfort and no local reaction at the site of injection.

CONCLUSION

This is not an ideal method because of the side-effects and the frequency of intramuscular injections required, but it is felt that at the present time intramuscular 15-me-PGF$_{2\alpha}$ with laminaria insertion and administration of antidiarrheals and antiemetics is an effective and safe method for termination of mid-trimester pregnancy. It is especially useful in patients with ruptured membranes, abortion failures by other methods and intrauterine fetal demise.

References

Berger, G. S. and Kerenyi, T. D. (1974a). Analysis of retained placenta saline abortions: methodologic considerations. *Am. J. Obstet. Gynecol.*, **120**, 479

Berger, G. S. and Kerenyi, T. D. (1974b). Analysis of retained placenta associated with saline abortion: clinical considerations. *Am. J. Obstet. Gynecol.*, **120**, 484

Berman, R., Hale, R. W., Reich, L. A. and Pion, R. J. (1974). Intra-amniotic prostaglandin PGF$_{2\alpha}$ (Tham salt) and the laminaria tent in midtrimester termination of pregnancy. *Contraception*, **9**, 635

Brenner, W. E., Hendricks, C. H., Dingfelder, J. and Staurovsky, L. (1973). Laminaria augmentation of intraamniotic prostaglandin F$_{2\alpha}$ for the induction of midtrimester abortion. *Prostaglandins*, **3**, 879

Bundy, G., Lincoln, F., Nelson, N. *et al.* (1971). Novel prostaglandin syntheses. *Ann. NY Acad. Sci.*, **180**, 76

Bygdeman, M., Martin, J. N., Wiqvist, N., Green, K., and Bergstrom, S. (1974). Reassessment of systemic administration of prostaglandins for induction of midtrimester abortion. *Prostaglandins*, **8**, 157

Bygdeman, M. and Wiqvist, N. (1971). Early abortion in the human. *Ann. NY Acad. Sci.*, **180**, 473

Corson, S. L. and Bolognese, R. J. (1979). Use of intramuscular 15(S)-15-methyl prostaglandin F$_{2\alpha}$ in failed abortions. *Am. J. Obstet. Gynecol.*, **133**, 145

Duenhoelter, J. H., Gant, N. F. and Jimenez, J. M. (1976). Concurrent use of prostaglandin F$_{2\alpha}$ and laminaria tents for induction of mid-trimester abortion. *Obstet. Gynecol.*, **47**, 469

Embrey, M. P. (1971). Induction of abortion by prostaglandin E (PGE$_1$ and PGE$_2$). *J. Reprod. Med.*, **6**, 256

Globus, M. S., Margolis, A. J., Sweet, R. L. and Laros, R. K. (1976). Experience with 276 intra-amniotic prostaglandin F$_{2\alpha}$ induced midtrimester abortions. *Prostaglandins*, **11**, 841

Green, K. and Bygdeman, M. (1977). Plasma levels of 15(S)-15-methyl PGF$_{2\alpha}$ following administration via various routes for induction of abortion. *Prostaglandins*, **14**, 1013

Gruber, W., Brenner, W. E., Stravrovsky, L. G., Dingfelder, J. R. and Wells, J. S. (1976). Evaluation of intramuscular 15(S)-15-methyl prostaglandin F$_{2\alpha}$ tromethamine salt for induction of abortion, medications to attenuate side effects, and intracervical laminaria tents. *Fertil. Steril.*, **27**, 1009

Karim, S. M. M. and Filshie, G. M. (1970). Therapeutic abortion using prostaglandin F$_{2\alpha}$. *Lancet*, **1**, 157

Karim, S. M. M. and Filshie, G. M. (1970): Use of prostaglandin E$_2$ for therapeutic abortion. *Br. Med. J.*, **1**, 198

Karim, S. M. M. and Sharma, S. D. (1972). Termination of second trimester pregnancy with 15 methyl analogues of prostaglandins E$_2$ and F$_{2\alpha}$. *J. Obstet. Gynaecol. Br. Commonw.*, **79**, 737

Lange, A. P. and Secher, N. J. (1977). Midtrimester and missed abortion treated with intramuscular 14(S)-15-methyl PGF$_{2\alpha}$. *Prostaglandins*, **14**, 389

Lauersen, N. H. and Wilson, K. H. (1975). Midtrimester abortion induced by serial intramuscular injections of 15(S)-15-methyl-prostaglandin F$_{2\alpha}$. *Am. J. Obstet. Gynecol.*, **121**, 273

Lauersen, N. H. and Wilson, K. H. (1977). The effects of intramuscular injections of 15(S)-15-methyl prostaglandin F$_{2\alpha}$ in failed abortions. *Fertil. Steril.*, **28**, 1044

Liggins, G. C. (1962). The treatment of missed abortion by high dosage. Syntocinon intravenous infusion. *J. Obstet. Gynaecol. Br. Commonw.*, **69**, 277

Lischke, J. H. and Goodlin, R. C. (1973). Use of laminaria tents with hypertonic saline amnioinfusion. *Am. J. Obstet. Gynecol.*, **116**, 586

Schwallie, P. C., Huang, D. C. and Turner, L. F. (1980). Use of intramuscular prostaglandin for failure of mid-trimester abortion by another method. *Contraception*, **22**, 623

Schwallie, P. C. and Lamborn, K. R. (1979). Induction of abortion by intramuscular administration of 15(S)-15-methyl PGF$_{2\alpha}$. *J. Reprod. Med.*, **23**, 289

Sharma, S. D., Hale, R. W. and Sato, N. E. (1975). Intramuscular 15(S)-15-methyl prostaglandin $F_{2\alpha}$ for midtrimester and missed abortions. *Obstet. Gynecol.*, **46**, 468

Southern, E. M., Gutknecht, G. D., Mohberg. N. R. and Edelman, D. A. (1978). Vaginal prostaglandin E_2 in the management of fetal intrauterine death. *Br. J. Obstet. Gynaecol.*, **85**, 437

Stubblefield, P. G., Naftolin, F., Frigoletto, F. D. and Ryan, K. J. (1974). Pretreatment with laminaria tents before mid-trimester abortion with intra-amniotic prostaglandin $F_{2\alpha}$. *Am. J. Obstet. Gynecol.*, **118**, 284

Stubblefield, P. G., Naftolin, F., Frigoletto, F. and Ryan, K. J. (1975). Laminaria augmentation of intra-amniotic $PGF_{2\alpha}$ for midtrimester pregnancy termination. *Prostaglandins*, **10**, 413

Stubblefield, P. G., Naftolin, F., Lee, E. Y. *et al.* (1976). Combination therapy for midtrimester abortion: laminaria and analogues of prostaglandins. *Contraception*, **13**, 723

WHO Task Force on the Use of Prostaglandins for the Regulation of Fertility (1977). Prostaglandins and abortion. I. Intramuscular administration of 15-methyl prostaglandin $F_{2\alpha}$ for induction of abortion in weeks 10 to 20 of pregnancy. *Am. J. Obstet. Gynecol.*, **129**, 593

Yankee, E. W. and Bundy, G. L. (1972). 15(S)-15-Methyl prostaglandins. *J. Am. Chem. Soc.*, **94**, 3651

11
Side-effects of natural prostaglandins

T. H. LIPPERT

INTRODUCTION

Although there is great interest in making clinical use of the diverse prostaglandin (PG) actions, it cannot be overlooked that they are also able to produce undesirable side-effects. Thus, it is important to recognize and be prepared for the pharmacological and toxicological actions of PGs in their therapeutic use.

While PGs have already been used routinely in obstetrics and gynecology for several years, they have now been introduced in other specialties such as pediatrics, radiology and internal medicine. Since most of the clinical work has been carried out with the natural PGs E and F, the following account is restricted to these drugs. In different organ systems their pharmacological actions are described and compared with side-effects observed during therapeutic use.

HEART AND CIRCULATORY SYSTEM

PGs can induce hemodynamic actions when large amounts reach the general circulation. High blood concentrations can arise due to inaccurate administration, e.g. in the uterine muscle instead of intended intra-amnial injection; also, after unusually good conditions for absorption or a deficient PG catabolism.

Table 11.1 summarizes the actions of PGE_2 and $PGF_{2\alpha}$ observed in humans and in several animal species (Eklund and Carlson, 1980; Malik and McGiff, 1976). With the exception of heart rate and cardiac minute volume, the type of reaction in other parameters is dependent on the particular PG administered. Thus, PGE_2 causes a fall in blood pressure with a simultaneous reduction in peripheral resistance. In contrast, $PGF_{2\alpha}$ increases blood pressure and peripheral resistance. With reduction in resistance of the coronary vessels due to PGE_2, improved circulation of the heart should result, whereas $PGF_{2\alpha}$ should have no action on the coronary vessels.

Generally the quantity of PG used therapeutically is less than that expected to produce a hemodynamic action. Apart from the very few lethal cases

Table 11.1 Actions of prostaglandins E_2 and $F_{2\alpha}$ on heart and circulatory system

	PGE_2	$PGF_{2\alpha}$
Heart rate	Increase	Increase
Minute volume	Increase	Increase
Blood pressure	Fall	Rise
Resistance of peripheral vessels	Decrease	Increase
Resistance of coronary vessels	Decrease	No observed action

reported, in which the circulatory system was always involved, there have been reports of a number of temporary hemodynamic side-effects. The circulatory changes did not appear in isolation but were usually associated with other systemic reactions. Influence on blood pressure and heart rate did not always correspond with the theoretically expected reaction. While after intravaginal and intra-amnial administration of PGE_2, a fall in blood pressure has been observed (Phelan et al., 1978; Ross and Whitehouse, 1974; Smith, 1974), unexpected decreases in blood pressure after $PGF_{2\alpha}$ have also been registered (Neeb, 1980; Ylöstalo et al., 1974). In addition, the heart rate was not only increased but a marked fall occurred after PGE_2 and $PGF_{2\alpha}$ (Fraser and Brash, 1974; Smith, 1974; Ylöstalo et al., 1974). The side-effects were usually minor and generally they were readily reversible. Doses of PGs were within the normal therapeutic range with the exception of one case (Smith, 1974). An overdose of 20 mg PGE_2 was given by intrauterine administration for hydatidiform mole. Since there are no fetal membranes in such a pregnancy, an intrauterine injection can be regarded as extra-amnial. Since the extra-amnial dose is not more than 200 μg if a gel formulation is not used, the dose given was 100 times greater (Karim, 1974). The severe shock which resulted could be controlled by symptomatic therapy only after 4 h.

An influence on local circulation by PG infusion has also been reported. Experiments have shown that PGE_2 increased circulation in the extremities while $PGF_{2\alpha}$ caused a decrease (Malik and McGiff, 1976). In a patient with a history of rubella arthropathy and since suffering from occasional numbness in the hands, 5–40 μg/min $PGF_{2\alpha}$ was infused for induction of labor in intrauterine fetal death (Roberts et al., 1972). The infusion had to be arrested because of cyanosis, loss of sensation in the hand and arm with decrease in skin temperature. Treatment was continued with oxytocin. Repetition of a $PGF_{2\alpha}$ infusion 3 months after the birth resulted in a similar reaction. The authors of this report suggest that the i.v. administration of $PGF_{2\alpha}$ is contraindicated in patients with a case history of peripheral vascular illness.

Burt et al. (1977) have reported the incidence of cardiac arrhythmia after $PGF_{2\alpha}$ administration. After 40 mg $PGF_{2\alpha}$ intra-amnially, weakness with fall in pulse and irregular heart rate occurred. Blood pressure remained uninfluenced at 120/80. The ECG showed frequent premature ventricular contractions with coupling bigeminy and trigeminy. These symptoms were connected with hypokalemia (2.8 mEq/l). In contrast to the above-mentioned hemodynamic side-effects, weakness appeared only 1 h after giving PG. The authors measured the potassium blood level in another 19 cases of PG-induced abortion and found a slight but significant fall. It was thought that the action of PG on electrolyte excretion by the kidneys was responsible for this effect. These investigators recommend that when the potassium blood level is already low, the use of PG should be contraindicated.

LUNGS

PGs play an important role in the lungs (Hyman *et al.*, 1978; Smith, 1976). Synthesizing and metabolizing enzymes for PGs are found in this organ in specially high concentrations. Besides physiological functions, the PGs are thought to be involved in illnesses such as asthma, lung embolism and lung oedema. Table 11.2 summarizes experimental results of function in humans and various animal species.

Table 11.2 Actions of prostaglandins E_2 and $F_{2\alpha}$ on the lungs

	PGE_2	$PGF_{2\alpha}$
Bronchial muscle	Relaxation (contraction also possible)	Contraction
Resistance of airways	Decrease (increase also possible)	Increase
Resistance of pulmonary vessels	Decrease (increase also possible)	Increase

In *in vitro* investigations PGE_2 caused relaxation of the human bronchial muscle while $PGF_{2\alpha}$ induced contractions. In *in vivo* examinations $PGF_{2\alpha}$ acted similarly, whereas E_2 induced bronchodilatation as well as broncho-constricting actions. Resistance of the airways always increased after $PGF_{2\alpha}$ while the reaction was inconsistent after E_2. Reversal of bronchodilatation to bronchoconstriction has been explained as due to metabolic processes of PGE_2 during the passage through the lungs. Present knowledge of the action on pulmonary circulation is based mainly on results of animal experiments. In these, $PGF_{2\alpha}$ caused vasoconstriction, while PGE_2 can cause vasodilatation or vasoconstriction.

The degree of reaction depends not only on the dose of PG administered but also on the mode of application. Intravenous infusion is less active than aerosol. In asthmatics the threshold is markedly lower than in healthy patients. The recognition of a danger to asthmatic patients has led to an examination of the influence of PGs on the lungs in healthy pregnant women. In five out of seven patients, signs of bronchoconstriction developed after PGE_2 infusions, 20 μg/min (Smith, 1973b). Following $PGF_{2\alpha}$ infusions, 200 μg/min, restricted pulmonary function was recorded in 13 of 19 pregnant patients (Smith, 1973b; Fishburne *et al.*, 1972). No changes in cardiac output, central venous pressure, blood pressure and heart rate were observed. In non-pregnant women a similar sensitivity of the lungs to PGs was apparent (Smith, 1973a).

It is astonishing that the number of published reports of pulmonary side-effects is relatively small. Single cases of bronchospasm in induction of abortion have been reported with the use of PGE_2 and $PGF_{2\alpha}$ (Anderson and Steege, 1975; Brenner et al., 1973; Fishburne et al., 1972; Fraser and Brash, 1974). PG was administered systemically and also locally in these cases. According to case history, a danger to the patient could not be anticipated in any case.

The influence of PG on pulmonary function should not affect the general condition of a healthy person. However, in a small group, e.g. asthmatics or chronic bronchitic patients in whom there is already restricted respiratory function, dramatic changes are possible. Thus it appears important that before PG is used, a case history of lung illness is sought and regarded as a contraindication to its use.

CENTRAL NERVOUS SYSTEM

PGs normally occur in the CNS and perform various functions, the mechanisms of which are still unknown (Coceani and Pace-Asciak, 1976). Generally they are associated with the modulation of cyclic nucleotides and neurotransmission. Also, due to changes in the cell membrane, ion permeability is altered. Table 11.3 shows some actions of PGs on the CNS as seen experimentally. Knowledge has been obtained mainly from animal experiments showing a marked sedative effect by PGE_2 while $PGF_{2\alpha}$ had no action, or only a very slight action. After intraventricular injection, the sedative action of PGE_2 is long-lasting but is of short duration after intravenous injection. Interesting, but not yet further examined, is the observation that PGs can influence the desire for food in animals (Baile et al., 1974). Cerebral circulation is inhibited by $PGF_{2\alpha}$ due to vasoconstriction. With PGE_2 vasodilatation and sometimes vasoconstriction has been observed. It is assumed that the particular effect depends on the requirements of individual regional areas. In humans, PGs are thought to play a role in pathological processes such as migraine and cerebral ischemia. The temperature-regulating centre in the hypothalamus reacts to PGE_2 and $PGF_{2\alpha}$ with a rise in temperature. This effect is similar to a pyrogen reaction; it differs in that only fever produced by PGs can be reduced by antipyretics of the aspirin type.

Table 11.3 Actions of prostaglandins E_2 and $F_{2\alpha}$ on the central nervous system

	PGE_2	$PGF_{2\alpha}$
Behavior	Sedation	No observed action
Cerebral vessels	Dilatation (contraction also possible)	Contraction
Body temperature	Increase	Increase

There are a number of publications concerning side-effects of PGs on the CNS. Reports of the incidence of epileptic seizures have led to examination of the EEG before and after PG (Faden *et al.*, 1976; Lyneham *et al.*, 1973; Shearman *et al.*, 1975; Van Der Plaetsen *et al.*, 1974). In up to 50 % of the patients examined, abnormal EEG curves were observed after $PGF_{2\alpha}$. However in induction of abortion with intra-amnial hypertonic saline, changes in the EEG were registered also. Therefore it is doubtful if this effect is a PG-specific one. There is a large discrepancy between the number of induced abnormal EEGs and incidence of seizures. The few cases of convulsions after PG were usually associated with untreated epilepsy. After PGE_2, as well as after $PGF_{2\alpha}$, convulsions were observed (Brash, 1976; Kaplan, 1978; Lyneham *et al.*, 1973; Shearmen *et al.*, 1975). However, in epileptic pregnant patients on anti-convulsive therapy, PGs did not induce convulsions (Fraser and Gray, 1974; MacKenzie *et al.*, 1973; Thiery *et al.*, 1974). Therefore danger of a seizure appears to be slight. Nevertheless, a case history of seizures in a patient should be a contraindication to the use of PG.

Disturbances of cerebral circulation after PG treatment have not been reported. Possibly headaches which often occur with PG-induced contractions are due to an influence on the blood vessels of various regions of the brain.

Rise in temperature due to PG occurs relatively often after PGE_2 and $PGF_{2\alpha}$. In most cases there is only a rise of $1-2°C$ but there are some reports of fever of $39-40°C$ and more (Phelan *et al.*, 1978; Smith, 1974). It is often difficult to show if a rise in temperature is a side-effect of PG or due to an infection. Especially in pregnancy termination, early recognition of an infection has important clinical consequences. Thus, it is recommended in patients with infection that PG should be avoided.

GASTROINTESTINAL TRACT

Under normal conditions, PGE_2 and $PGF_{2\alpha}$ occur in the gastrointestinal tract. In the intestine especially there is an efficient enzyme catabolic system, so that after oral administration only small quantities can reach the systemic circulation. According to many investigators the PGs play an important role in various physiological and pathophysiological functions in the gastrointestinal tract (Bennett, 1976). Table 11.4 summarizes various actions of exogenous PGs.

Table 11.4 Actions of prostaglandins E_2 and $F_{2\alpha}$ on the gastrointestinal tract

	PGE_2	$PGF_{2\alpha}$
Secretion of acid gastric juice	Inhibition	No observed action
Secretion of intestinal juice	Stimulation	Stimulation
Passage through small intestine	Accelerated	Accelerated
Intestinal motility	Inhibition (stimulation also possible)	Stimulation (inhibition also possible)

The influence on gastric secretion has aroused special interest with the hope that PGE_2 or an E_2 derivative might inhibit hyper-secretion of the gastric glands. This inhibitory effect can only be seen after i.v. administration as PGE_2 is only slightly absorbed by the mucosa. Newer derivatives, however, are also active orally. $PGF_{2\alpha}$ did not inhibit gastric secretion. The action of PGE_2 and $PGF_{2\alpha}$ on intestinal secretion is well documented (Robert, 1976). The mechanism consists of a reduction of water and electrolyte absorption by the intestine with simultaneous stimulation of water and electrolyte secretion in the intestinal lumen. The fluid which accumulates in the small intestine is excreted as diarrhea, speeding up passage in the small intestine. Both oral and parenteral PG can cause this effect.

Generally, PGE_2 inhibits intestinal motility and $PGF_{2\alpha}$ leads to stimulation. Species differences and varying results between *in vitro* and *in vivo* results, in which PGE_2 also causes stimulation and $PGF_{2\alpha}$ relaxation, have led to a confused picture.

In the therapeutic use of PG, the gastrointestinal side-effects play a dominant role. Diarrhea is caused by both types of PG and, according to frequency of occurrence, this is a peak for side-effects; although the percentage varies widely from author to author, this effect is mentioned in almost every publication. Since in induction of abortion, i.v. administration of PG produced diarrhea with nausea and vomiting in up to 100 % of the cases, local administration with a lower incidence of side-effects is used. Thus, gastrointestinal side-effects have been reduced markedly but not totally eliminated. Increased intestinal motility resulting in intestinal cramps has also been reported (Hunt *et al.*, 1975). Although these side-effects are not serious for healthy patients, they nevertheless reduce the acceptance of prostaglandins.

UTERUS

The occurrence of primary PGs in endometrium and in the decidua of the uterus has led to linking this with the physiology and pathophysiology of menstruation and onset of birth (Karim and Hillier, 1975; Lippert, 1977). The precise mechanism of action in initiating labor is not yet clear. Interactions with cyclic nucleotides and intracellular calcium mobilization probably play a role. There are indications that there is a direct effect of PG on the muscle cells.

Table 11.5 shows the *in vivo* actions of primary PGE_2 and $PGF_{2\alpha}$ on the uterus of pregnant and non-pregnant women.

Table 11.5 Actions of prostaglandins E_2 and $F_{2\alpha}$ on the uterus

	PGE_2	$PGF_{2\alpha}$
Non-pregnant uterus	Relaxation (contraction also possible)	Contraction
Pregnant uterus	Contraction	Contraction

134

Exogenous PGE_2 causes relaxation in the non-pregnant uterus at menstruation and also at ovulation (Bygdeman *et al.*, 1979; Toppozada *et al.*, 1975). At other stages in the cycle it causes contractions. $PGF_{2\alpha}$ induces contractions at all times in both the pregnant and non-pregnant uterus. At ovulation, however, uterine sensitivity to $PGF_{2\alpha}$ appears to be reduced. In sufficiently high doses both PGs are able to induce contractions at any stage of pregnancy, resembling spontaneous contractions at term.

The initial effect depends on the speed of administration. When injection is rapid there is a temporary increase in basal tone, while with slower administration the basal tone remains unchanged. There are a number of publications concerning side-effects of PGs on the uterus. Non-specific complications such as infection after local application, mechanical injury due to curettage or bleeding after incomplete expulsion of the placenta are not considered. These effects are not specific for PGs but also occur after other methods of induction of abortion. However, the high uterine activity can lead to uterine damage, especially to cervical injury (Fraser, 1974; Göretzlehner and Klausch, 1974; Kajanoja *et al.*, 1974; Lowensohn and Ballard, 1974; Perry *et al.*, 1977; Purandare *et al.*, 1977). These occurred after PGE_2 and $PGF_{2\alpha}$ using various modes of administration. The incidence is specially high when additional medication with oxytocin was given, as is done when uterine contractions are good but the cervix remains tense and non-dilated. This type of damage is almost exclusively seen in primiparas. Perry and co-workers (1977) have suggested the different mechanisms for cervical dilatation in primi- and multiparas as responsible. In addition to so-called transverse tears which can lead to complete detachment of the cervix, longitudinal tears have also been reported. Usually the injuries do not produce severe bleeding and symptoms of shock do not appear. Thus it is possible to overlook cervical injury if post-examination is omitted. Surgical care is not always simple and in some cases a cervicovaginal fistula is residual. Cervical injury has been recorded using other methods for interruption of pregnancy but the frequency of $1-3\%$ with PGs is higher.

A late complication after PG abortion is the increased incidence of spontaneous abortion in later pregnancies, possibly due to cervical insufficiency (MacKenzie and Hillier, 1977). However, according to other investigations, the frequency of cervical insufficiency after PG abortion is not unusually high (Embrey, 1975).

Another very serious side-effect of PG treatment is uterine rupture (Borten and Friedman, 1978: Bromham and Anderson, 1980; McCarthy and McQueen, 1980; Sandler *et al.*, 1979). The incidence is markedly smaller than the incidence of cervical laceration. As with induction by oxytocin, multigravid women present a specially high risk. Patients with myoma or previous cesarean section are also at danger. Tears have been described in each part of the corpus. With severe hemorrhage the patient is in acute danger and in most cases hysterectomy is necessary.

In induction of labor at term, the incidence of uterine hypertony has been reported (Roberts and Turnbull, 1971). The danger appears to be specially great when PGE_2 tablets are given. However, Thiery and Amy (1976) contradicted this opinion and reported that oral administration is not more hazardous than i.v. infusion. According to these authors the occurrence of nausea may be considered a warning that the therapeutic dose has been exceeded.

BLOOD COAGULATION

Normally, PGE_2 and $PGF_{2\alpha}$ are liberated by platelets during the process of coagulation. It is still not clear what role the primary PGs play in this process (Howie, 1976). Initially it was suspected that only the precursors, the PG-endoperoxides, were functional in coagulation. Now it is known that prostacyclin and thromboxane A_2, derived from endoperoxides, are involved in coagulation (Moncada et al., 1980). Of the primary PGs only PGE_1 can influence platelet function significantly. It has a marked inhibitory effect on aggregation, and after thrombus formation it accelerates disaggregation.

When PGE_2 and $PGF_{2\alpha}$ are given therapeutically their influence on coagulation is weak or insignificant (Howie, 1976). In the use of PGs for interruption of pregnancy there have been no reports of coagulation disturbance of clinical importance. Hemorrhage after expulsion of the fetus is generally slight.

SKIN

It was observed that increased PG concentration was present in exudate from skin injuries caused by burns, eczema or UV radiation, and so it was thought that PG might play a role in inflammatory reactions in the skin (Greaves, 1976; Lewis, 1975). PGE_2 causes an increase in vessel permeability, whereas $PGF_{2\alpha}$ antagonizes this effect, producing oedema and erythema, with liberation of other inflammatory substances such as histamine and brady-kinin. Pain and itchiness may not be due to a direct PGE_2 action in inflammatory reactions. However the actions of histamine, bradykinin and other factors are probably potentiated by PGE_2.

Frequently, production of erythema around the infusion needle has been observed (Smith and Mason, 1974). When the infusion is withdrawn this side-effect disappears again quickly.

MORTALITY

During the early years of clinical use it was thought that PGs provide a less complicated therapy than other substances, especially when used for termination of pregnancy in the second trimester. A large number of cases had to be reviewed before some of the serious complications became apparent. In the meantime there have been reports of mortality which are linked with the use of PGs. Termination of advanced pregnancy is in itself a potential risk, and it is to be expected that serious complications can occasionally arise. A number of fatalities have occurred during PG treatment. In the literature available, there are reports of ten fatal cases, nine of which occurred with $PGF_{2\alpha}$ and one with PGE_2 (Cates *et al.*, 1977; Cates and Jordaan, 1979; Haller and Kubli, 1978; Patterson *et al.*, 1979). An analysis shows that in seven cases the PG participation in the fatal outcome was only marginal. In the remaining three cases, in which $PGF_{2\alpha}$ was given intra-amnially, it is assumed that the PG was directly responsible for the fatal outcome.

Symptoms shortly after administration of PG, e.g. vomiting, respiratory distress, headache, gastric cramp and seizures with collapse, are actions of PGs which can be observed experimentally in the various organs.

These reports should make it clear that while the use of PG is considered as safe, there is occasionally the risk of serious complications arising. However, immediate treatment of recognized complications should enable prevention of the side-effects developing to a dangerous extent.

References

Anderson, G. G. and Steege, J. F. (1975). Clinical experience using intraamniotic prostaglandin $F_{2\alpha}$ for midtrimester abortion in 600 patients. *Obstet. Gynecol.*, **46**, 591

Baile, C. A., Martin, F. H., Forbes, J. M., Webb, R. L. and Kingsbury, W. (1974). Intrahypothalamic injections of prostaglandins and prostaglandin antagonists and feeding in sheep. *J. Dairy Sci.*, **57**, 81

Bennett, A. (1976). Prostaglandins and the alimentary tract. In Karim, S. M. M. (ed.). *Prostaglandins: Physiological, Pharmacological and Pathological Aspects.* p. 247. (Lancaster: MTP Press)

Borten, M. and Friedman, E. A. (1978). Uterine rupture: a complication of midtrimester abortion. *Prostaglandins*, **15**, 187

Brash, J. H. (1976). A generalized epileptiform convulsion after intra-amniotic prostaglandin E_2. *Br. J. Obstet. Gynaecol.*, **83**, 665

Brenner, W. E., Dingfelder, J. R., Hendricks, C. H. and Staurovsky, L. G. (1973). Introduction of therapeutic abortion with a single dose of intra-amniotically administered prostaglandin $F_{2\alpha}$. *Prostaglandins*, **4**, 485

Bromham, D. R. and Anderson, R. S. (1980). Uterine scar rupture in labour induced with vaginal prostaglandin E_2. *Lancet*, **2**, 485

Burt, R. L., Connor, E. D. and Davidson, I. W. F. (1977). Hypokalemia and cardiac arrhythmia associated with prostaglandin-induced abortion. *Obstet. Gynecol.*, **50**, 45

Bygdeman, M., Bremme, K., Gillespie, A. and Lundström, V. (1979). Effects of the prostaglandins on the uterus. *Acta Obstet. Gynecol. Scand.*, Suppl. **87**, 33

Cates, W. and Jordaan, H. V. F. (1979). Sudden collapse and death of women obtaining abortions induced with prostaglandin $F_{2\alpha}$. *Am. J. Obstet. Gynecol.*, **133**, 398

Cates, W., Grimes, D. A., Haber, R. J. and Tyler, C. W. (1977). Abortion death associates with the use of prostaglandin $F_{2\alpha}$. *Am. J. Obstet. Gynecol.*, **127**, 219

Coceani, F. and Pace-Asciak, C. R. (1976). Prostaglandins and the central nervous system. In Karim, S. M. M. (ed.). *Prostaglandins: Physiological Pharmacological and Pathological Aspects.* p. 1 (Lancaster: MTP Press)

Eklund, B. and Carlson, L. A. (1980). Central and peripheral circulatory effects and metabolic effects of different prostaglandins given i.v. to man. *Prostaglandins*, **20**, 333

Embrey, M. P. (1975). Prostaglandin-induced Abortion and Cervical Incompetence. *Br. Med. J.*, **2**, 497

Faden, A., Golbus, M. S. and Spire, J. P. (1976) Electroencephalographic changes following intraamniotic prostaglandin $F_{2\alpha}$ administration for therapeutic abortion. *Obstet. Gynecol.*, **47**, 607

Fishburne, J. I., Brenner, W. E., Braaksma, J. T., Staurovsky, L. G. Mueller, R. A., Hoffer, J. L. and Hendricks, C. H. (1972). Cardiovascular and respiratory responses to intravenous infusion of prostaglandin $F_{2\alpha}$ in the pregnant woman. *Am. J. Obstet. Gynecol.*, **114**, 765

Fraser, I. S. (1974). Complications of Prostaglandin-induced Abortion. *Br. Med. J.*, **4**, 404

Fraser, I. S. and Brash, J. H. (1974). Comparison of extra- and intra-amniotic prostaglandins for therapeutic abortion. *Obstet. Gynecol.*, **43**, 97

Fraser, I. S. and Gray, C. (1974). Prostaglandin $F_{2\alpha}$ and electroencephalogram changes. *Lancet*, **2**, 49

Göretzlehner, A. and Klausch, B. (1974). Transverse posterior cervical rupture following extra-amniotic prostaglandin $F_{2\alpha}$-induced abortion. *Am. J. Obstet. Gynecol.*, **119**, 865

Greaves, M. W. (1976). Prostaglandins and inflammation. In Karim, S. M. M. (ed.). *Prostaglandins: Physiological, Pharmacological and Pathological Aspects.* p. 293. (Lancaster: MTP Press)

Haller, U. and Kubli, F. (1978). Klinische Nebenwirkungen und Komplikationen der Prostaglandine bei Abortinduktion. *Gynäkologie*, **11**, 39

Howie, P. W. (1976). Prostaglandins and blood-coagulation. In Karim, S. M. M. (ed.). *Prostaglandins: Physiological, Pharmacological and Pathological Aspects.* p. 277. (Lancaster: MTP Press)

Hunt, R. H., Dilawari, J. B. and Misiewicz, J. J. (1975). The effect of intravenous prostaglandin $F_{2\alpha}$ and E_2 on the motility of the sigmoid colon. *Gut*, **16**, 47

Hyman, A. L., Spannhake, E. W. and Kadowitz, P. J. (1978). Prostaglandins and the lung. *Am. Rev. Resp. Dis.*, **117**, 111

Kajanoja, P., Jungner, G., Wildholm, O., Karjalainen, O. and Seppälä, M. (1974). Rupture of the cervix in prostaglandin abortions. *J. Obstet. Gynaecol. Br. Commonw.*, **81**, 242

Kaplan, E. (1978). A generalized epileptiform convulsion after intra-amniotic prostaglandin with intravenous oxytocin infusion: a case report. *S. Afr. Med. J.*, **53**, 27

Karim, S. M. M. (1974). Adverse reactions to intra-amniotic prostaglandin. *Br. Med. J.*, **3**, 347

Karim, S. M. M. and Hillier, K. (1975). Physiological roles and pharmacological actions of prostaglandins in relation to human reproduction. In Karim, S. M. M. (ed.). *Prostaglandins and Reproduction.* p. 23. (Lancaster: MTP Press)

Lewis, G. P. (1975). *The Role of Prostaglandins in Inflammation.* p. 161. (Bern: Hans Huber Publishers)

Lippert, T. H. (1977). Die Prostaglandine in der reproduktiven Physiologie. *Klin. Wochenschr.*, **55**, 515

Lowensohn, R. and Ballard, C. A, (1974). Cervicovaginal fistula: an apparent increased incidence with prostaglandin $F_{2\alpha}$. *Am. J. Obstet. Gynecol.*, **119**, 1057

Lyneham, R. C., McLeod, J. G., Smith, I. D., Low, P. A., Shearman, R. P. and Korda, A. R. (1973). Convulsions and electroencephalogram abnormalities after intra-amniotic prostaglandin $F_{2\alpha}$. *Lancet*, **2**, 1003

MacKenzie, I. Z. and Hillier, K. (1977). Prostaglandin-induced abortion and outcome of subsequent pregnancies: a prospective controlled study. *Br. Med. J.*, **2**, 1114

MacKenzie, I. Z., Hillier, K. and Embrey, M. P. (1973). Convulsions and prostaglandin-induced abortion. *Lancet*, **2**, 1323

Malik, K. U. and McGiff, J. C. (1976). Cardiovascular Actions of Prostaglandins. In Karim, S. M. M. (ed.). *Prostaglandins: Physiological, Pharmacological and Pathological Aspects.* p. 103 (Lancaster: MTP Press)

McCarthy, T. and McQueen, J. (1980). Uterine rupture as a complication of second trimester abortion using intraamniotic prostaglandin E_2 and augmentation with other oxytocic agents. *Prostaglandins*, **19**, 849

Moncada, S., Flower, R. J. and Vane, J. R. (1980). Prostaglandins, prostacyclin and thromboxane A_2. In Goodman, L. S. and Gilman, A. (eds.). *The Pharmacological Basis of Therapeutics.* p. 668 (New York: Macmillan)

Neeb, U. (1980). Wirksamkeit und Nebenwirkungen der intrazervikalen Prostaglandin $F_{2\alpha}$-Gel Applikation im 1.Trimenon. *Geburtsh.u.Frauenheilk.*, **40**, 901

Patterson, S. P., White, J. H. and Reaves, E. M. (1979). A maternal death associated with prostaglandin E_2. *Obstet. Gynecol.*, **54**, 123

Perry, G., Siegal, B. and Held, B. (1977). Uterine trauma associated with midtrimester abortion induced by intra-amniotic prostaglandin $F_{2\alpha}$, with and without concomitant use of oxytocin. *Prostaglandins*, **13**, 1147

Phelan, J. P., Meguiar, R. V., Matey, D. and Newman, C. (1978). Dramatic pyrexic and cardiovascular response to intravaginal prostaglandin E_2. *Am. J. Obstet. Gynecol.*, **132**, 28

Purandare, V. N., Ganguli, A. C., Gharse, R. M. and Krishna, U. R. (1977). Cervico-vaginal injuries in cases of second trimester termination of pregnancy. *Prostaglandins*, **13**, 349

Robert, A. (1976). Antisecretory, antiulcer, cytoprotective and diarrheogenic properties of prostaglandins. In Samuelsson B. and Paoletti, R. (eds.). *Advances in Prostaglandin and Thromboxane Research*, Vol. 2, p. 507. (New York: Raven Press)

Roberts, G. and Turnbull, A. C. (1971). Uterine hypertonus during labour induced by prostaglandins. *Br. Med. J.*, **1**, 702

Roberts, G., Mottram, R. F., Parry, H and Bloom, A (1972). Cyanosis due to intravenous prostaglandin $F_{2\alpha}$. *Lancet*, **2**, 425

Ross, A. H. and Whitehouse, W. L. (1974). Adverse reactions to intra-amniotic urea and prostaglandin. *Br. Med. J.*, **1**, 642

Sandler, R. Z., Knutzen, V. K., Milano, C. M. and Gleicher, N. (1979). Uterine rupture with the use of vaginal prostaglandin E_2 suppositories. *Am. J. Obstet. Gynecol.*, **134**, 348

Shearman, R. P., Lyneham, R. C., Walsh, J. C. Itzkowic, D. and Shutt, D. A. (1975). Elektroencephalographic changes after intraamniotic prostaglandin $F_{2\alpha}$ and hypertonic saline. *Br. J. Obstet. Gynaecol.*, **82**, 314

Smith, A. M. (1974). Adverse reactions to intra-amniotic prostaglandin. *Br. Med. J.*, **2**, 382

Smith, A. P. (1973a). Side-effects of prostaglandins. *Lancet*, **2**, 655

Smith, A. P. (1973b). The effects of intravenous infusion of graded doses of prostaglandins $F_{2\alpha}$ and E_2 on lung resistance in patients undergoing termination of pregnancy. *Clin. Sci.*, **44**, 17

Smith, A. P. (1976). Prostaglandins and the Respiratory System. In Karim, S. M. M. (ed.). *Prostaglandins: Physiological, Pharmacological and Pathological Aspects.* p. 83 (Lancaster: MTP Press)

Smith, E. R. and Mason, M. M. (1974). Toxicology of the prostaglandins. *Prostaglandins*, **7**, 247

Thiery, M. and Amy, J. J. (1976). Uterine hypertonus after induction of labour with prostaglandin E_2 tablets. *Br. Med. J.*, **1**, 958

Thiery, M., Amy, J. J., Hemptinne de D. and Yo Le Sian (1974). Prostaglandins and convulsions. *Lancet*, **1**, 218

Toppozada, M., Gaafar, A., Shaala, S. and Osman, M. (1975). The relaxant property of local prostaglandin E_2 on the non-pregnant uterus – a cyclic response. *Prostaglandins*, **9**, 475

Van Der Plaetsen, L., Thiery, M., Amy, J. J. and Hemptinne de D. (1974). Effect of prostaglandin E_2 therapy on the cerebral cortex. *Lancet*, **1**, 1226

Ylöstalo, P., Kauppila, E. and Vapaatalo, H. (1974). Complications following the intra-amniotic administration of prostaglandin $F_{2\alpha}$ for therapeutic abortion. *Acta Obstet. Gynecol. Scand.*, **53**, 279

12
Epilogue

E. S. E. HAFEZ

BIOCHEMICAL PARAMETERS

Prostaglandins, 20-carbon unsaturated fatty acids, are formed by enzymatic oxidation and cyclization of certain essential fatty acids (Figs 12.1–12.4). The main precursor of bio-unsaturated prostaglandins is arachidonic acid, found in the 2-position of cell membrane phospholipids which is liberated in response to certain stimuli by a lysosomal enzyme (Figs 12.4 and 12.5). In the presence of molecular oxygen and numerous microsomal enzymes, arachidonic acid is converted into labile endoperoxides G_2 and H_2.

Some glycerophospholipids of the amnion and chorion, namely *phosphatidylethanolamines*, are particularly rich in arachidonic acid. The placental membranes possess a phospholipase A_2 specific for phosphatidyl-ethanolamines (Okazaki *et al.*, 1978).

Prostaglandins possess specific membrane-binding sites. They are not

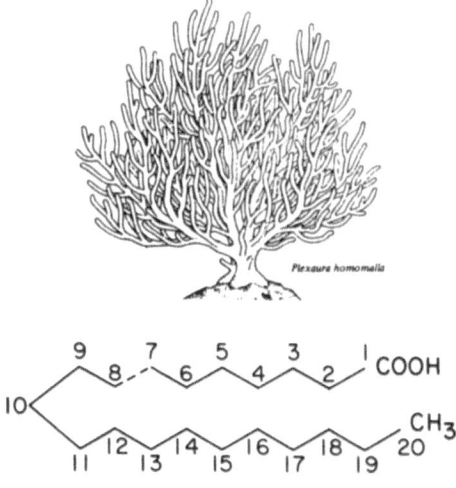

Figure 12.1 Basic structure of prostanoic acid, the theoretic 20-carbon molecule with a cyclopentane ring, which is common to all natural prostaglandins (Dingfelder, 1980)

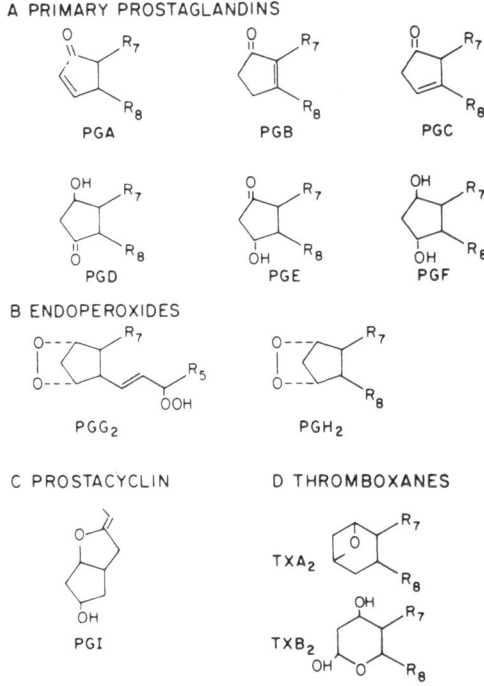

Figure 12.2 Ring structures of primary prostaglandins, endoperoxide intermediates, and prostacyclin and thromboxane derivatives. Note that thromboxanes have 6-carbon rings whereas all other structures have 5-carbon rings. (Dingfelder, 1980)

antagonized by antihistamines, atropine, serotonin antagonists, alpha- or beta-blocking agents, or oxytocin antagonists (Amy *et al.*, 1984).

PHYSIOLOGICAL PARAMETERS

Naturally occurring prostaglandins perform various physiological functions, and cause numerous pharmacological effects on the different segments of the reproductive tract. Some of these physiological mechanisms include: release of pituitary gonadotropins, ovarian and testicular steroidogenesis, ovulation, gamete transport and implantation.

Once synthesized in chorion and decidua, prostanoids are transported, probably by diffusion, into the myometrium, which is being activated, and into the amniotic fluid, causing higher titers (Amy and Karim, 1978). During active labor, mechanical disturbance and hypoxia may augment the release of certain enzymes controlling the synthesis of prostanoids, thus making myometrial contractility a self-perpetuating phenomenon (Amy *et al.*, 1984). Prostanoids derived from arachidonic acid have major physiological functions such as softening and dilatation of the cervix (Calder, 1979), activation

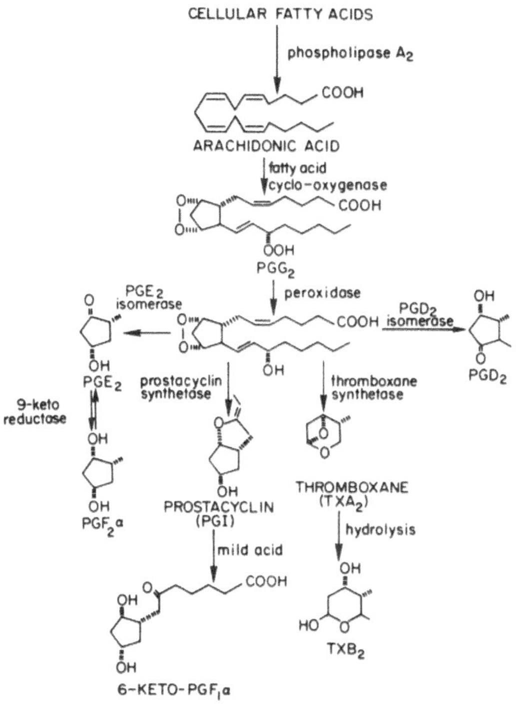

CELLULAR FATTY ACIDS

phospholipase A_2

COOH

ARACHIDONIC ACID

fatty acid cyclo-oxygenase

COOH

OOH

PGG_2

peroxidase

PGE₂ isomerase

PGD_2 isomerase

COOH

OH

PGE₂ isomerase

9-keto reductase

OH

PGE_2

prostacyclin synthetase

thromboxane synthetase

OH

PGD_2

OH

OH

$PGF_2\alpha$

PROSTACYCLIN (PGI)

THROMBOXANE (TXA_2)

hydrolysis

mild acid

COOH

OH

OH

OH

HO

TXB_2

OH

6-KETO-$PGF_1\alpha$

Figure 12.3 Overall scheme of formation of prostaglandins, prostacyclins, and thromboxanes from fatty acid precursors and endoperoxide intermediates (PGG_2 and PGH_2). Selective inhibition of the various enzymes listed is possible and may permit accumulation of greater or lesser amounts of various end products. (Dingfelder, 1980)

of the myometrium and expulsion of the conceptus throughout all stages of pregnancy (Liggins *et al.*, 1977). Inhibitors of prostaglandin synthesis suppress myometrial activity and thereby, depending on the timing of administration, postpone and/or prolong labor (Keirse, 1979; Amy & Thiery, 1980).

The sensitivity of the myometrium to PGF_2 or PGE_2 varies throughout the menstrual cycle, being more sensitive in the proliferative and secretory phases than around the time of ovulation. The sensitivity of the myometrium to $PGF_{2\alpha}$ and PGE_2 decreases after the administration of oral contraceptives. The hypercontractility pattern experienced during dysmenorrheic episodes may be due to increased synthesis of $PGF_{2\alpha}$.

The non-pregnant cervix contains densely packed finely wavy collagen fibers. During pregnancy the fibers in the cervical waves are broader and deeper. The administration of prostaglandins causes similar changes when some bunched fibers split into fibrils with a periodicity of $640 \, \text{Å}$ which is typical for collagen.

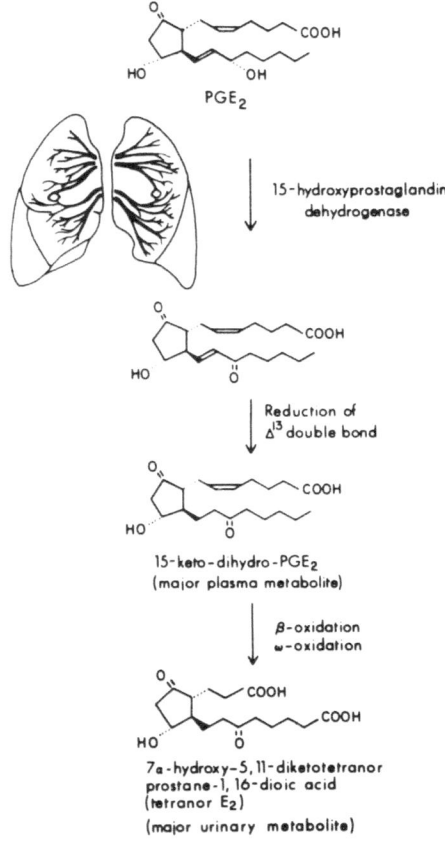

PGE_2

15-hydroxyprostaglandin dehydrogenase

Reduction of Δ^{13} double bond

15-keto-dihydro-PGE_2
(major plasma metabolite)

β-oxidation
ω-oxidation

7α-hydroxy-5,11-diketotetranor prostane-1, 16-dioic acid
(tetranor E_2)
(major urinary metabolite)

Figure 12.4 Body metabolism of a primary prostaglandin. Conversion to plasma metabolite occurs within minutes, therefore metabolite values will more nearly reflect ongoing metabolism than will measurement of primary prostaglandins. Tetranor urinary metabolite is useful for following prostaglandin metabolism over a number of hours or days. (Dingfelder, 1980)

EVALUATION OF PG ANALOGS

A variety of prostaglandin analogs used as abortifacients have been extensively tested to evaluate optimal doses, vehicles and routes and intervals for administration. The metabolism and pharmacokinetics of 15-methyl-$PGF_{2\alpha}$ have been studied following intravenous, intra-amniotic, intramuscular and vaginal administration. Various formulations of 9-deoxo-16,16-dimethyl-9-methylene are used for early and late first trimester abortion and for menstrual induction.

Extensive investigations were done to evaluate the potency and activity of PGs in softening and dilating the uterine cervix. Attempts to separate the uterine-stimulating effects of prostaglandins from a direct action on the cervix

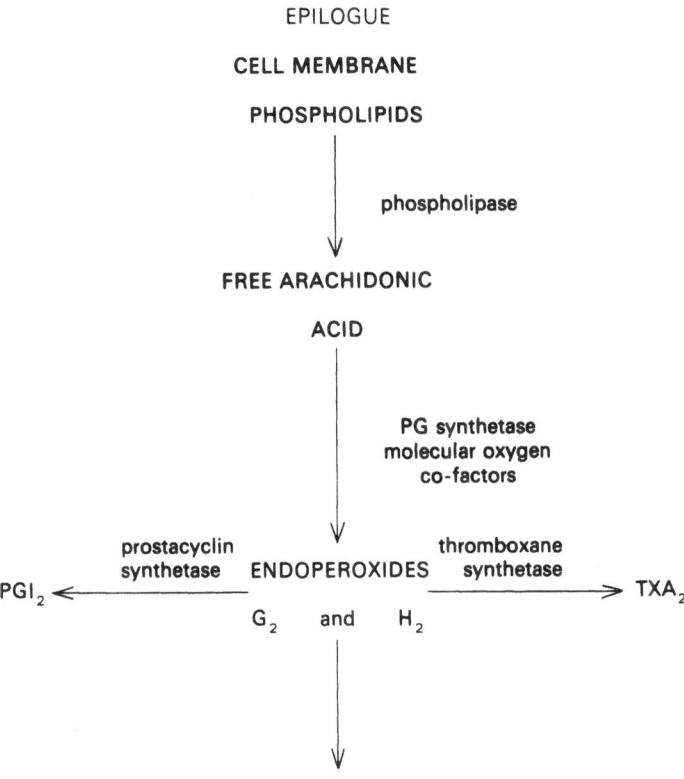

Figure 12.5 Simplified scheme of the 'arachidonic acid cascade' (biosynthesis of prostanoids). (Amy *et al.*, 1984)

have prompted studies on the biochemical changes in the cervix during spontaneous and induced cervical dilation.

Two functional units are recognized in the uterus: muscular segment; and lower segments, composed primarily of connective tissue. Prostaglandins interfere with the connective tissue within the cervical stroma, which is abundantly innervated by monoaminergic nerves utilizing norepinephrine as a transmitter. This causes remarkable changes in the biophysical and biochemical characteristics of the cervix.

Several research attempts have been made towards the development of precise drug delivery by means of laminated polymeric membrane systems. This was accomplished by the judicious selection of membranes with optimal permeability characteristics to achieve a wide range of zero-order release rates. The laminated delivery module consists of a non-permeable support membrane, a drug-bearing membrane, and an outer membrane which controls the rate of prostaglandin release.

PROSTAGLANDINS FOR ABORTION

Mechanical dilatation of the cervix preceding voluntary interruption of pregnancy can cause trauma to the cervix. Complications from forceful dilatation include immediate tissue damage to the cervix (laceration and creation of false passages), cervical incompetence, and future premature delivery and spontaneous abortion. Prostaglandins and their analogs, with prolonged action and reduced side-effects, soften and change the rigidity of the cervix. Naturally occurring prostaglandins, because of their rapid metabolism, inactivation and associated gastrointestinal side-effects, are less suited for preoperative dilatation.

In several countries, mid-trimester abortion has been induced by the intra- or extra-amniotic administration of prostaglandins, as well as by intra- muscular and vaginal administration. The effectiveness of prostaglandins in inducing second trimester abortion varies with parity; stage of gestation; pretreatment Bishop score; and the type, dosage and route of prostaglandin administration. There are marked differences in the reported rate of successful inductions, degree of side-effects, and the induction–abortion interval. It may be possible to facilitate the provision of abortion service by developing an analog which can be self-administered in the outpatient department or at home.

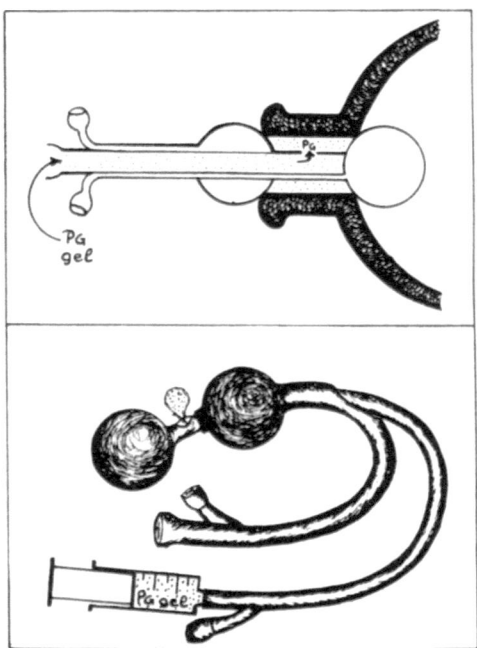

Figure 12.6 *Bottom*: Cervical catheter. *Top*: Administering PG gel into cervical canal (designed by Dr. T. Tsalikis)

146

Mode of administration

These compounds have been employed using various routes of administration and formulations: intramuscular, vaginal, intracervical, intra-amniotic, extra-amniotic and intravenous; using solutions, suppositories or tablets. 'Tsalikis catheter' is used to overcome the difficulties of local application of prostaglandins into the cervical canal. This catheter consists of two Folley's catheters; the smaller of which is inserted into the larger. After the insertion of this cervical catheter, the inner balloon closes the internal os firmly and the outer presses the external os. After the inflation of the balloons, prostaglandin is inserted into the cervical canal, in divided doses, at regular intervals.

Side-effects

Prostaglandins stimulate gastrointestinal contractility and have variable effects on body temperature, bronchial muscles and blood pressure. The use of prostaglandins to induce abortion may cause several complications such as rupture of the uterus and disseminated intravascular coagulation (Table 12.1). However, whether these are PG-specific, related to the abortion process or due to concomitant use of different therapeutic agents remains to be evaluated.

Table 12.1 Deaths associated with abortion by intra-amniotic administration of a prostaglandin

Compound	Pre-existing conditions	Cause of death
$PGF_{2\alpha}$[a]	Chronic alcoholism; pancreatitis; pontine myelolysis	Hematemesis + aspiration
$PGF_{2\alpha}$[a]	Severe congestive heart failure	?? Amniotic fluid embolism
$PGF_{2\alpha}$[a]	Chronic hypertension; severe superimposed pre-eclampsia	Hypertensive crisis + cerebral hemorrhage
$PGF_{2\alpha}$[a]	—	Intravenous narcotic + phenothiazine; respiratory arrest
Intravenous oxytocin + intra-amniotic NaCl + intra-amniotic $PGF_{2\alpha}$[a]	—	Septicemia; DIC; acute tubular necrosis
$PGF_{2\alpha} + NaCl$[b]	—	Septicemia; hemolysis or DIC
$PGF_{2\alpha}$[c]	Grand multiparity	Uterine rupture; shock, death during hysterectomy
15-methyl-$PGF_{2\alpha}$[c]	Grand multiparity	Delayed post-abortal bleeding (day 12); shock; death during hysterectomy

[a] Cates *et al.*, 1977; [b] Adachi *et al.*, 1977; [c] Tejuja *et al.*, 1978

Various pharmacological responses have been reported following PGE_2 and $PGF_{2\alpha}$ administration, such as: inhibition of gastric acid secretion; stimulation of water and electrolytes in small intestines; restricted respiratory function and even bronchospasm in individual cases. $PGE_{2\alpha}$ causes contraction of bronchial muscles and constriction of brain vessels. Body temperature is raised by both PGE_2 and $PGF_{2\alpha}$ by central stimulation. In induction of abortion there have been some incidences of epileptic seizures, increased temperature and headache.

OTHER CLINICAL USES OF PGs

Prostaglandin suppositories are effective for post-conception menstrul induction (menstrual regulation). If cost, availability and stability factors are favorable, prostaglandins can successfully compete with extraction and expulsion techniques to induce abortion throughout gestation.

Compounds which inhibit prostaglandin synthesis, or which modulate other specific steps in the arachidonic acid cascade, have been extensively used in the treatment of dysmenorrhea, premature labor, endometriosis, dysfunctional and IUD-induced uterine bleeding, and toxemia of pregnancy.

The uterine-stimulating activity of prostaglandins has been utilized to terminate viable and non-viable pregnancies, and to treat refractory cases of atomic postpartum hemorrhage. Thus, prostaglandins seem to be more effective than other oxytoxic agents for pregnancy termination at the early stages of gestation and for avoiding problems associated with abnormal pregnancy and term labor. Low doses of prostaglandins have been used to facilitate the insertion of intrauterine devices.

In rodents and domestic animals several prostaglandin analogs cause luteolysis and disruption of the estrous cycle or early pregnancy. These effects were utilized under farm conditions for the synchronization of estrous cycles for artificial insemination, super-ovulation and subsequent embryo transfer.

References

Adachi, A., Wilson, L. and Herzig, N. (1977). Prostaglandin F2 hypertonic saline and oxytocin in midtrimester abortion. *N.Y. State J. Med.*, **77**, 46

Amy, J., Brucker, P. and Merckx, M. (1984). Control of uterine activity in pregnancy. In Hafez, E. S. E. (ed.). *Spontaneous Abortion* (Boston: MTP Press)

Amy, J. J. and Karim, S. M. M. (1978). Prostaglandins and other oxytocic substances in amniotic fluid. In Fairweather, D. V. I. and Eskes, T. K. A. B. (eds.). *Amniotic Fluid – Research and Clinical Application*, 2nd edn, pp. 321–345. (Amsterdam: Excerpta Medica)

Amy, J. J. and Thiery, M. (1980). Labor – spontaneous and induced. In Aladjem, S., Brown, A. K. and Sureau, C. (eds.) *Clinical Perinatology.* pp. 362–381. (St. Louis: C. V. Mosby)

Calder, A. A. (1979). Management of the unripe cervix. In Keirse, M. J. N. C., Anderson, A. B. M. and Bennebroek-Gravenhorst, J. (eds.) *Human Parturition.* pp. 201–217. (Leiden: University Press)

Cates, W., Jr., Grimes, D. A., Haber, R. J. and Tyler, C. W., Jr. (1977). Abortion deaths associated with the use of prostaglandin $F_{2\alpha}$. *Am. J. Obstet. Gynecol.*, **127**, 219–231

Dingfelder, J. R. (1980). Prostaglandins. In Hafez, E. S. E. (ed.). *Human Reproduction, Conception and Contraception,* 2nd edn. pp. 727–729. (Hagerstown: Harper & Row)

Keirse, M. J. N. C. (1979). Prostaglandines et declenchement spontane du travail. In Amy, J. J. (ed.) *Les Prostaglandines et la Reproduction Humaine.* pp. 107–140 (Paris: Flammarion Medecine-Sciences)

Liggins, J. C., Forster, C. S., Grieves, S. A. and Schwartz, A. L. (1977). Control of parturition in man. *Biol. Reprod.,* **16,** 39

Okazaki, T., Okita, J. R., MacDonald, P. C. and Johnson, J. M. (1978). Initiation of human parturition. X. Substrate specificity of phospholipase A_2 in human fetal membranes. *Am. J. Obstet. Gynecol.,* **130,** 432

Tejuja, S., Choudhury, S. D. and Manchanda, P. K. (1978). Use of intra- and extra-amniotic prostaglandins for the termination of pregnancies – reports of multicentric trial in India. *Contraception,* **18,** 641–652

Index